Brent W. Robinson

Dianomics™

The Economics of Diabetes

A Powerful Economic Strategy for Disease Prevention and Treatment

Brent W. Robinson, M.B.A.

Library of Congress Cataloging-in-Publication Data
Robinson, Brent W., 1957-
Dianomics™: The Economics of Diabetes. A powerful economic strategy
for disease prevention and treatment.
Includes References
ISBN-13: 978-1470157654
1. Patient health incentives. 2. Diabetes treatment and prevention
3. Healthcare reform.
Printed in the United States of America
Cover design by Debbie Seigler, Design Studio 7

DEDICATION

To all those suffering with obesity

Important:

All opinions expressed and policy recommendations herein are the sole responsibility of the author and do not reflect the opinion or policy of The Diabetes Economist Inc., or the Institute for Health and Productivity Management (IHPM).

This work is not an official publication of IHPM.

The stories and examples herein are illustrative only, and do not refer to any specific living or deceased individuals.

This publication is intended to provide general information regarding the direct and indirect costs of diabetes. It is not intended to provide financial, medical or dietary advice, counsel, or opinion for any individuals or their families. It is the understanding of the author, as expressed throughout the work that all readers will seek direction from a licensed accounting professional and medical provider for all financial, dietary and medical needs.

This work, including all references, does not recommend or endorse any specific tests, medical providers, products, procedures, opinions, websites, or other professional services or information.

CONTENTS

Σ

The "cure" for the diabetes epidemic will not be found in the science of medicine, it will be found in the science of economics.

As assuredly as wealth is driving the epidemic of diabetes, wealth can halt it. Financial incentives created to support our healthy behavior will allow us to conquer diabetes.

Author
June 2012

ACKNOWLEDGMENTS

My deepest gratitude and appreciation extends to my family, friends and colleagues for their support of this work. Without their unflinching encouragement this book would still be in the cradle of imagination. My parents Stephen L. Robinson and Marion Robinson provided their expert editing and review. My wife Debbie and our children Stephanie and husband Matthew, Scott and wife Chari, Benjamin and Joshua supplied extensive editing, research assistance, critique, and insight. My thanks also to my colleagues within the pharmaceutical, healthcare, and workforce productivity industries; all of them work tirelessly to find solutions for patients suffering from chronic diseases. Kudos to book covers design expert Debbie S., and proof reader Cassandra, who assisted with the creative and editing processes.

Brent W. Robinson

Σ

INTRODUCTION

Millions are dying each year from the complications of diabetes and obesity. Diabetes and obesity advance in spite of all prevention efforts. The world's most enlightened scientists and physicians have yet to find a cure or a reasonable solution to preventing the spread of diabetes throughout developing countries. By 2050, one in three of us will be dealing directly with the effects of this deadly pandemic plague. For hundreds of years, the world searched in vain for the cure of the vicious bubonic plague. Claims were made that the plague was due to God's wrath and that trying to stop the ravages of the illness were beyond the control of mere mortals. Wives' tale cures, sorcery spells, and priestly prayers all proved to be no match for the almighty flea and microscopic bacteria.

Anciently, we did not comprehend how disease is transmitted via unseen bacteria. Now, every physician comprehends bacterial illnesses, as well as why diabetes and obesity develop. Although most patients do not know that overeating on a regular basis destroys vital organs, physicians have proved, and we understand, that overeating makes us fat. We also know that it is extremely challenging to stop overeating. In attempting this feat, the majority of us have tried and failed.

To eliminate the diabetes and obesity pandemic, we must stop eating so much. Eating less is not a matter of willpower. It is not a matter of our genes. It is not a matter of more education. It is not a matter of medical science. Eating less is a matter of motivation. We have little or no motivation in our culture to eat less. Instead, we have the opposite: the ability to eat more, much more than we need. The balance of motivation is way off, in favor of readily available high fat, sugary and salty foods. The balance of motivation is not on our side. From this imbalance, most of us are directly or indirectly losing ground both physically and financially. This imbalance leaves us with a stark choice. We can follow our current path to oblivion by eating too much or we can find a power in our environment strong enough to change our motivation, and swing us back into balance. *Dianomics* is a book about finding that balance once again by unleashing and harnessing a motivating power great enough to prevent the ravages of diabetes and obesity.

This motivating power is found in the driving force of all developing countries – personal economic incentives. *Dianomics* helps us understand that it is the power of economics that may help us avoid overeating. Economic power shapes our lives and directs us to where we can live, where we can work, what we can wear, what car we can drive, what college we can attend, and even whom we can date. The economic powers preventing us from contracting diabetes and obesity are slumbering dormant in our homes, at our schools, with our employer, and throughout our healthcare systems. Personal economic incentives surround us, and are waiting to be embraced. These incentives shape our daily decisions and can be utilized to create a healthier life, a life free from diabetes and obesity, a life free from over eating, a life free from our plague.

Within the pages of *Dianomics*, we uncover a treasure trove of powerful motivations and economic incentives designed to encourage our healthy behaviors. These incentives are treasures because they add to our collective health and wealth. They do not cost any more money. They can be found by anyone willing to dig for them. Now, they are no longer hidden, patented or protected. These treasures are the precious personal solutions for the diabetes and obesity epidemic. *Dianomics* seeks to bring them to life by offering them to the public for scrutiny and debate.

These economic motivators, our treasures, are readily found in our homes, ethnic communities, schools, workplaces and healthcare systems. The home is a place where older children can earn allowance for healthy eating and activity. Home is a place where parents can lead by example and put to use their financial resources to secure their healthy eating habits. Home is also a place where a culture of incentives can be born.

Schools can be financially motivated to implement a public health policy that quantifies the epidemic and identifies at-risk children and their parents. Through legislating incentives into law, governments can support schools in their efforts to protect at-risk children and control the spread of the disease. At school, children, with their parents, can receive screening and powerful motivation to engage in healthy activity and nutritious diets. They can be taught the financial penalties and physical consequences of failure in the fight against obesity.

Ethnic communities stand to win big-time by deploying the incentive treasures found in *Dianomics*. These communities, the fastest growing segment of our society, have children that are disproportionately threatened by the epidemic due to a grossly improper diet, unsafe neighborhoods, weak education, and a lack of substantial incentives. Personal responsibility health initiatives, culturally appropriate education, and new property tax incentives can be introduced at little or no cost and can address these serious challenges inherent in our minority cultures.

Clearly, maximizing our health through incentives at work is an excellent investment for businesses. Employers have the power of insurance at their beck and call. Insurance designs can be transformed into a motivational platform that coaches employees and uncovers health risks. *Dianomics* suggests that health insurance design can reinforce compliance to our doctors' prescribed personal treatment plan, improve health outcomes, and reduce healthcare expenses. Based on our productivity, employers know our level of health, and can reward our healthy choices accordingly.

Physicians and hospitals are currently incentivized to practice national quality guidelines and to refrain from excessive tests and procedures. Fully implementing these guidelines will free up resources, enabling our healthcare system to more effectively and forcefully focus on disease prevention. Compensating physicians for helping the poor produces greater access to care for our underserved populations. Physician incentive compensation can also prevent grandma and grandpa from dying needlessly in pain and discomfort in the hospital. As explained in *Dianomics*, grandma and grandpa would rather die at home with the assistance of hospice care, surrounded by their loved ones. Physicians, with proper encouragement, can ensure that our seniors pass on with dignity and grace.

Medicare, the institution protecting our seniors, and the most likely of all our health care systems to go bankrupt, can unleash economic incentives to restore fiscal normalcy. *Dianomics* explains how to do this without raising taxes. Medicare can incentivize the development of end-of-life patient directives and change the incentives for physicians such that no longer will one out of ten seniors receive an operation in the last week of life. Medicare can heal itself with proper changes—incentives that reward patient responsibility and appropriate provider interventions.

Highlighted within the pages of *Dianomics* is the understanding that personal economic health incentives are powerful enough to change the course of a disease. They are powerful enough to end an epidemic. Uncovering, examining, testing, and implementing these incentives is the mission of this work. It may come as a revelation to the public, as well as to the medical community, that personalized economic incentives are effective and ready for deployment. This revelation will cause a rethinking of our healthcare priorities in a manner that redirects scarce resources towards supporting greater personal responsibility. Personalized financial incentives will change the way our culture approaches the treatment and cure for diabetes and obesity. The economic principles of *Dianomics* may pave the way for us to understand our personal responsibilities in ending the most costly and deadly pandemic of our generation. *Dianomics* is a treasure, a powerful economic strategy for disease prevention and treatment.

$$\Sigma$$

CHAPTER 1

BETA CELLS

Wake up America - and the world! Our beta cells are dying! And no one is telling you! You and I have beta cells in our bodies that are critical for life, and they are dying at a faster rate than ever before. Here is an indisputable fact about our bodies: if we overeat most of the time and become fat, <u>we burn out our pancreatic beta cells prematurely</u> and become a person with diabetes. Our scientists suggest that by the time a child or an adult is first diagnosed with type 2 diabetes, they may have already lost 50% of their pancreatic beta cell function (Butler et al. 102-10). Premature beta cell death from chronic overeating is almost universally preventable.

Diabetes is a very serious disease with severe morbidity and high mortality rates. How is it that every man, woman, and child does not know this vital information about the death of beta cells, and that it is what causes diabetes to occur in our bodies? After spending 25 years associated with the diabetes medical community, it remains perplexing to me that this fact is not understood by the general public. The concept is as simple as "cigarettes cause cancer", or as straightforward as, 'don't drink and drive, because if you do you will cause death and destruction." In fact, if you chronically over-eat, beta cell death is more certain than being hit by a drunk driver! Beta cell burnout is irrefutably linked to an early and painful death. Why are we not dealing with it in these terms?

"It's the economy stupid!"(Attributed: to James Carville from the 1992 Presidential campaign for Bill Clinton)

The answer is simple, economics. The economic incentives in our culture, intended to help us avoid this disabling and deadly disease, are simply not strong enough, or are non-existent altogether. Misaligned economics saturate our culture—from our families and employers to our insurance companies and governmental agencies. No one has applied the powerful financial tools necessary to help us modify our eating behavior. As a result, we have created the most costly, most sugary, and fattiest epidemic in the history of the world.

Having sold the world's leading diabetes products, including insulin, for decades, I came to the conclusion that although medicine initially controls patient blood sugar levels, the medicine in and of itself does nothing to change a patient's behavior over the long term. This unchanged behavior is the root cause of the disease. I witnessed firsthand that doctors are helpless to prevent costs and manage diabetes effectively over the long run, because physicians cannot change chronic overeating patterns, nor reverse the loss of healthy beta cells.

Patient behavior is the key to solving our beta cell loss epidemic–not medicine. Physicians are really powerless to eliminate the underlying causes of the disease. Let's break it down this way: If I receive a gift of $500,000 dollars, will I use some or all of it? Yes (if taxes don't take it first!). I would rush out and buy my first car, or home, or pay off my student loans. No law against that. How about this: what if I live in the wealthiest country in the history of the world, full of every conceivable combination of delicious and rich foods, will I eat them? Of course I will–especially if I still have my $500,000 of free money, after I pay off my student loans. I, along with most people, will spend my gifted money, and dine like the kings and queens of old.

But here is the rub–what if I spend the money on vice and drugs, not food and fun? Then I turn around and make a mess of my life, such that my actions cost you $500,000 of your money to clean up my life. 'Not so fair!' you say. And, what if I overeat myself into a disease that costs you and others $500,000 dollars of your money to try and save me? Surprisingly, right now our answer is, "That's ok, and it is well within his or her rights. Let them eat away! Eat, drink and be merry, for tomorrow may never come."

So, we rightly ask the question: what expected economic disincentive is there for someone to be powerfully persuaded to stop expecting other citizens' money and possessions? Now consider our beta cell burnout epidemic. Our perceived expectant cost for overeating is minimal. We have absolutely no concept of what economic consequences await us if we continue our risky behavior; just floating vagaries about future "possible risks", like we are reading an investment statement. Furthermore, children are uniformly unable to conceive of the economic burden of overeating and certainly cannot understand that they may be eating their way into developing a chronic disease that can bankrupt their future.

Let us return to my prize winnings of $500,000. Can I, or any person, through our long-term food indulgences, incur costs in the healthcare system of $500,000? If so, perhaps I need to *forfeit my $500,000 prize* in lieu of my impending healthcare costs. After all, I may spend my money on food and vice, so now my healthcare costs fall to my friends, family, employer, as well as my beloved fellow citizens to cover. This is truly the sobering reality. If you are 50 right now, and become diagnosed with diabetes, it will cost, on average, $170,000 to treat you for life, assuming you take care of yourself (Zhuo).

The lifetime cost to treat someone who is diagnosed today at age 30 is on average $300,000 for their lifetime. Who will pay for the nearly 100,000,000 Americans that will be diagnosed with diabetes by the year 2050? (CDC Division of Media Relations) We have established that for someone diagnosed today between 30 and 50 years of age, it will cost the healthcare system approximately $150,000 to $300,000 over their lifetime. Because we are living longer, and utilizing more expensive procedures to treat our medical complications, we can expect total costs to treat diabetes to double or triple over the next 25 years. (Rabin)

If we are diagnosed at age 30 in 2035, the lifetime cost to treat our diabetes will be $500,000 or close to a half of million dollars! So, here I am, your $500,000 friend who just turned 25. Because of my poor eating habits, I unfortunately become a patient with diabetes on my 50th birthday. I can expect you, my friends, family, and fellow citizens to help me pay my expected $500,000 dollars in direct lifetime medical care. Thank you very much. The cake was worth it. And I ate it.

Economic Incentives

Clearly lacking are the economic incentives in our culture that impact us, our families, and our friends in ways that protect us from permanently killing our beta cells. Physicians can diagnose and extend all the excellent support and resources they have to offer. In the end we are quickly overwhelmed by our environment and do not follow our physician's advice. We are even told that not changing course may mean possible dire medical consequences. Yet the half-million dollar scenario we just discussed plays out over and over again. <u>Our personal willpower is no match for our incredibly abundant food choices and eating opportunities.</u>

As a society, and as individuals, we simply do not understand the importance of owning the financial impact of our poor nutritional choices. Nor have we reinforced our environment and culture to deal with this deficit in a way that adequately protects our children. The alarming fact is that children who develop type 2 diabetes face tremendous lifetime implications that include greater risks for eye, kidney, and heart disease, as well as greater probability of stoke, obesity, cancer, and possibly lower fertility and income. To prove this point, please consider the following statistic.

Chapter 1

Table 1

Financial Impact of Patients with Diabetes

American Diabetes Association Statistics

(Diabetes Care 31:596-615, 2008 and the National Diabetes Fact Sheet)

Financial Impact for patients with diabetes:

1. Medical expenses are 2.3 time higher
2. Heart Disease death rate is 2-4 times higher
3. Leading cause of blindness
4. Leading cause of kidney failure
5. Leading cause of amputation
6. $1 in $5 is spent on caring for someone with diabetes

(Centers for Disease Control and Prevention)

Children and adults who develop diabetes are, because of the disease's effects, less productive at work than their healthy counterparts. Their current and future employers will pay thousands of dollars more for their medical costs. The other significant medical reality is that type 2 diabetes in children (and adults) is completely preventable, and was hardly ever diagnosed 30 years ago. (U.S.Department of Health and Human Services)

This book offers numerous solutions to this challenge. But first, it examines the untold and unthinkable economic risks confronting us and our children, and dishes them out in a heaping proportion to make the death of our beta cells up front and personal. You will see clearly, by the end of your investigation, your personal responsibility in the matter, and what the severe financial implications are for all of our over-consumption. You will see how you can play a role in creating the solutions to this problem. You will find what it takes to thwart the disease progression in our culture, and how we may save our future generation as a result of embracing and implementing these vital changes.

What is up with these Beta Cells?

The beta cells reside on the pancreas and are stimulated by sugar to produce insulin. When too much sugar is ingested two important events occur. Firstly, over time, our beta cells burn out (think of a heart attack where if we artificially raced the heart for 20 years we would burn out our heart muscles cells). Secondly, as the body tries to respond to all of this excessive sugar from overeating, over time, too much insulin is produced. Too much insulin and too much sugar in the body cause our cells to resist the effects of insulin, and we develop insulin resistance. Our bodies simply cannot take it anymore. Our cells begin to refuse to process the sugar and insulin normally.

Consider this example. Once a water reservoir is full, where do we put the rest of the water? It is the same with our bodies. We have already stored the extra calories as fat everywhere on our bodies (just look down and pinch your stomach). We have no more use for the extra food; however, we cannot simply turn off the spigot like we can do with the water reservoir, because our mouths stay wide open. The excess food begins to burn out our beta cells and shut down our body's capacity to use insulin and sugar as originally designed. The long term result of all of this overeating is that we become unable to produce the energy we need to survive. We become a person with type 2 diabetes.

Note: To be clear, certain diabetes, less than 10%, occurs spontaneously, and is not caused by chronic overeating. Due to unknown causes, or perhaps an infection or an inappropriate immune response, the beta cells in some of us simply stop producing insulin. This is termed type 1 diabetes, and occurs primarily in children. <u>Type 1 diabetes is not caused by overeating and is thought to be a condition that is not generally preventable. A discussion around economic incentives for preventing type 1 diabetes is wholly inappropriate.</u> As with all of us, the proper management of our sugar and overall calorie intake is paramount to good health and to long life, including those of us with type 1 diabetes

<u>Children in Jeopardy</u>

Our children's health is in grave danger. The CDC reports that by the year 2050 one in three of all Americans will have burned out some portion of their beta cells and become diagnosed with diabetes. That means, on average, one person in every American family that is a child now will develop diabetes! If you have three children, one will, on average, be diagnosed. This statistic is not farfetched. Currently, in some age groups the rate for obesity is one in six already. Obesity caused by overeating and inactivity is directly relatable to the incidence of diabetes.

Chapter 1

Table 2

<u>Prevalence of Obesity</u>

Please examine the rates of obesity at: Data from NHANES surveys (1976–1980 and 2003–2006) (Centers for Disease

Control and Prevention) showing that the prevalence of obesity has doubled or tripled:

- for children aged 2–5 years, prevalence increased from 5.0% to 12.4%;
- for those aged 6–11 years, prevalence increased from 6.5% to 17.0%;
- and for those aged 12–19 years, prevalence increased from 5.0% to 17.6%

The ramifications of this are astounding. This disease trend suggests that diabetes and obesity will evolve into the direct or indirect leading killer of the next generation. The proof of this rising threat can be seen in the alarming rise of obesity and the accompanying diagnosis of type 2 diabetes in our school age children. The most current data suggests that two million children ages 12-19 have pre-diabetes.(Centers for Disease Control and Prevention)

Economic Importance of Beta Cells

If insulin is so important to our health, why is the message of beta cell burnout so nonexistent in our culture, media, and national dialogue? The answer: because it is economically irrelevant to the common man. It means nothing. There is no compelling motivation to the upside or downside of our chronic overeating. Let the French fries fall where they may – or let the sugary drinks flow into the belly of our kids - it doesn't matter. We collectively think, "What is it costing me now – and besides my kids are happy."

To reiterate, if we are a relatively healthy 30 year old now, but are overeating regularly and continue to do so until we are diagnosed with diabetes at age 50, we may cost the medical system in the US an estimated $500,000 over our lifetime, just to help us with our lack of beta cells. If dynamic economic incentives are not introduced, diabetes has the potential to bankrupt our medical system, our employer-sponsored insurance industry, and our retirement systems.

Our most dedicated physicians, excellent diabetes educators and brilliant drug discovery scientists cannot save us from the end of this rainbow. There will not be a pot of gold there – only an ocean of manmade insulin and syringes. Why insulin? Because, as physicians can rightly tell us, if we live long enough, most patients with diabetes will lose their remaining insulin-producing beta cells over time and will need insulin injections to survive. In the meantime, what options do doctors have to work with? This may surprise you.

Treating the Epidemic – Our Current Solutions

Before mentioning the following options, please keep in mind that all patients with diabetes must be closely monitored and report their calories and activity to their healthcare providers. This is a preeminent and necessary approach to maintaining their health. Also, please keep in mind that the research scientists' economic incentive is to find aids that cause the pancreas to keep producing insulin so patients can live normal lives.

Diabetes Product Categories

In reviewing drugs for diabetes, ask yourself this question: are any of these agents designed to *help produce more* beta cells? Actually, I will save you the trouble; the answer is no. To do so would be the equivalent of taking a pill or shot that rebuilds arteries and heart tissue after a heart attack. No drug on the market does that either.

Note:

If you are prescribed any of these products, do not under any circumstance stop taking your prescribed medicine. Continue to take your prescribed medicine exactly as you have been instructed by your healthcare provider. If you have any questions, see your pharmacist or healthcare provider. Always follow your physician's recommendations. This section is written only to assist you in understanding the mode of action of each category of product. Consult your health care professional with any questions.

Chapter 1
Table 3
Product Categories to Treat Diabetes
(Oral Diabetes Medications)

1. Biguinides – One of the most widely studied and recommended products. Their action reduces the amount of stored and circulating glucose, so the body can attempt to function normally. Metformin does not directly cause the body to produce more beta cells

2. Sulfonylureas – The most widely used category of agents historically, and one of the oldest know treatments for diabetes. Action – stimulates the remaining beta cells to secrete more insulin. These products do not create more beta cells.

3. Meglitinides – Stimulates functioning beta cells to secrete insulin (similar to Sulfonylureas), but in a blood

glucose dependent fashion. These products do not create more beta cells.

4. Alpha-glucosidase Inhibitors - inhibit glucose absorption from the intestines. These products do not produce more beta cells.

5. Thiazolidinediones (TZD's) - Improve the way the body uses insulin by reducing insulin resistance in patients with diabetes. These agents do not help the body produce more beta cells.

6. DPP-4 inhibitors. Increases insulin secretion and decreases the amount of glucose that the liver produces. These products do not directly produce more beta cells.

7. GLP-1 Increases insulin production in response to meals and decreases the amount of glucose that the liver produces. It also slows the emptying of food from the stomach.

8. Insulin – Insulin, in its many commercially available forms, attempts to replace naturally occurring human insulin. External insulin has not been shown to create new beta cells.

So there you have it--all the main modern medicine categories used to treat diabetes. We learn something stunning from this review. Over the last decades, the amount of research dollars spent on finding treatments for diabetes exceeds tens of billions of dollars. The excellent primary research conducted by almost all of the largest pharmaceutical companies in the world has produced agents that only modulate glucose and insulin. True, these wonderfully talented scientists created the world's finest products. We applaud them, and thank them from the bottom of our hearts. These valuable medicines have prolonged lives, improved health, and increased the quality of lives of hundreds of millions of people around the world.

Little, if any, of the profits derived from the sales of these products go directly to the development of procedures or *products that assist the body in growing new beta cells.* To be fair, no one knows if regenerating any body organ is feasible, except perhaps through stem cell manipulation and implantation. Certainly, it can be said that there is no product that can grow back all of the beta cells that are killed off in the course of developing diabetes. It is not yet possible to accomplish this feat through pharmaceuticals.

From a business point of view, what percentage of profit is directed to finding an actual cure for diabetes? Are pharmaceutical companies investing in possible treatments or are they motivating their scientists to be the first to *cure* the disease? There simply is little economic benefit for them to cure the disease at this point in the epidemic, because they earn a lot more money treating a disease then curing one. Bottom line: do not expect a cure anytime soon—at least from the pharmaceutical industry.

The cure for type 2 diabetes is behavioral. We will need a cultural event the size of a major earthquake to set us on the right path. This huge shift needs to be the size of the 1962 Alaska earthquake: the second largest earthquake in recorded history, and the most powerful one recorded on U.S. soil. It had a magnitude of 9.2.

Let the cultural shift begin, and let it begin with my child

The diabetes epidemic problem with children is ground zero for change. Remember the fact that type 2 diabetes in children is almost completely preventable. Every child needs to know about the power of insulin, and the importance of beta cells. They also need to experience the economic incentives in their culture that motivate positive nutrition and healthy activity. The following section outlines numerous activities for parents, children, schools, and governments to follow to begin shaping incentives that have the potential to change our children's behavior over the long term.

Do children understand that there are economic consequences for not avoiding diabetes? <u>Not likely, since we have established the fact that most adults do not have a robust understanding themselves, and this lack of understanding may follow them for the remainder of their lives</u>.

What follows are solutions to this issue at the individual child level. These ideas are offered not as proven incentives for behavior change, but as a means to begin the dialogue and to interject economic principles that can drive cultural change and individual behavior. Let us examine mild financial interventions first, followed by more aggressive strategies, through the story of Johnny, a young 10 year old boy living in the southern United States. Although what you will read next about Johnny's behavior and his environment is not real, the science behind the story is formulated on proven economic principles.

Johnny's Story

Johnny is a great kid. He loves his parents and they love him. Johnny had a problem. He loved eating sweets. He gained way too much weight for his age according to his pediatrician, the family's longtime, trusted doctor. The more weight he gained the less active he became, and so on. So, his parents decided to help him out. They agreed to give Johnny a substantial allowance. Johnny liked this idea because he was saving for his first bicycle.

As with any allowance, Johnny had to earn it. At the beginning of each week, Johnny got his allowance. During the week, he was active for an hour a day and only ate sweets on the weekends. When he did this, he got the allowance again at the beginning of the next week. Johnny began to be successful, his weight began to decrease, and his energy level improved. He began to exercise every day and stopped eating sweets, except on the weekends. He eventually earned enough money to buy the bicycle. Johnny's parents decided this program would be good for them as well, so they made the same allowance rules for themselves. They did it as a family. Now, the family goes for bike rides on the weekends.

Parents can help a child reach important health goals by establishing financial incentives. Although this is a simple example and may not work in every situation, it teaches us that working with a child in their home environment, with incentives that are really important to the child, produce healthy results. The results are improved if parents participate in the incentive. (For additional information on home based incentives for children needing to eat better and exercise more, see Appendix Table 1, 2, 3).

As Johnny progressed, the parents asked themselves, "I wonder what Johnny is eating at school? Johnny spends so much of the day there." The parents investigated and were pleasantly surprised. They realized that their son's school had a good understanding of childhood health and nutrition.

Supporting our Children's Nutritional Goals in a School Environment

The parents in Johnny's school district had learned about the very real danger of children growing up in a poor nutrition (high fat/salt/sugar), low activity (excessive TV watching, computer gaming) world. They took matters into their own hands and got approval from the school board to implement impactful education with incentives to support themselves and their children. They quickly realized that they could not be successful without the guidance of their wonderful teachers, administrators, and volunteers. The following is a fantastic example of how Johnny's school community backed up one another and especially helped children just like Johnny.

Although Johnny was not a lover of tests, especially on the first day of class, he nonetheless put his head down and started reading. What he was reading was interesting to him, so he did not mind the short quiz that followed. The subject was on health, and it taught him about his beta cells. He never even knew he had a pancreas, let alone these special cells that were important to protect because they helped his body create the energy he needed. He found out that his parents were right, that if he ate poorly and was not active, he could actually be damaging his health. He was glad he found this out early on in school. It helped him understand why the school acted the way they did about lunch menu choices and physical education.

"What" Johnny did not see happening behind the scene was the other part to the story. His parents were participating in the test as well. They had agreed with the school board that this education should start in third grade, and be given each year, all the way through college, in a format that was appropriate to the age group. <u>Not only that, the parents agreed to bear the full responsibility for the completion of the questionnaire</u>. They agreed to require all students, third grade through college, to submit the completed questionnaire within 60 days of starting each school year. They decided that the test or questionnaire could be completed either online, at school, by mobile phone, by land line, by text message, by a class volunteer, by fax, during school, by the PTA, <u>or by any other method approved</u> by the school district. They removed any and all logistical reasons why a parent could not help their child complete the assignment. Then, the earthquake hit. Boom! It was the incentive that made it all mean something.

There were important incentives added. The school collected a $5.00 fee to administer this education. A child's guardian was fined 30 dollars a month up to 200 dollars in any given school year if the questionnaire was not completed within the first 60 days of school attendance. There were added incentives. Completion of the questionnaire was part of the qualifications for children participating in the free school lunch program. To further motivate the kids, test completion qualified them to win the chance to help select special items from the pre-approved school lunch menu.

A New State Law

What came next? Well, let us just say it took a while to get used to.... The parents in Johnny's school district agreed to follow the new state law. The new law based on health statistics identified obesity in children and young adults as an epidemic. And indeed, it fit the definition well. An epidemic is something that "[adversely] affects a disproportionately large number of individuals within a community at the same time." Diabetes and childhood obesity rates were at an all-time high in their area.

To impact this trend, a plan was agreed upon. It went something like this (for complete details see Chapter 1 Appendix Table 4, 5): students in the state were weighed and their body mass index (BMI) calculated (all statistics were kept confidential). Students who were in a high risk category for diabetes/obesity (as established by national guidelines) were automatically enrolled along with a guardian, in nutrition, beta cell protection, and activity education. All costs (approximately $90) for the education of these at risk children were the responsibility of their respective parent or guardian. Learning from history, the state realized that there must be incentives for compliance. Penalties up to $200 for failure to complete the prescribed education within 60 days were applied. This seemed harsh, but it proved to be vital to achieving compliance.

Johnny found that his BMI placed him squarely in the high risk category, so he and his family completed the education. His Dad completed it grudgingly. He hated the idea that the school was asking him to do it, but he was bound and determined to avoid paying the fine for something that was designed to help his family. The education itself was powerful. It included a 5 part series that described how obesity could affect the family's future employment and health (including amputation, blindness, cancer, and infertility, to name a few). After completing the education, the family agreed that the allowance program they had started together with Johnny was really well worth every penny. What surprised Johnny's dad even more was the new Federal law that the states needed to comply with in order to receive help with the epidemic. We will call this the aftershock.

Federal Law (example) – the Epidemic Zone

The state Johnny's family was living in had incredible costs associated with obesity and diabetes. The U.S. Congress passed legislation that helped address the proven epidemic. The new federal law required establishing Epidemic Zones (EZ) for areas with high obesity rates. (See Chapter 1 Appendix Table 6) The full name of the zones was Beta Cell Endangerment Zones (BCEZ), and was designed specifically to protect children. Johnny and his family, as it turns out, were getting educated on how the epidemic was affecting their family because of the amount of Medicaid and Medicare dollars the federal government was spending in their community, specifically on the health of chronically overeating citizens and their dependents.

Once Johnny's dad heard about the program, he was impressed and thought it was a good use of his tax dollars. This is what he found out: BSEZ's are identified by where children are at the greatest risk, based on weight statistics. Each school in the state must record and submit the number of children at risk for diabetes or obesity. Each BCEZ school must submit a parent-approved plan to assist all children attending the high risk schools. This plan enables the community to understand the importance both economically and medically of staying physically fit.

This had a profound effect on Johnny's mother because her own mother had recently prematurely died from complications of diabetes, and she herself had gained a lot of weight since Johnny's birth. She found out that physical examinations were automatically scheduled for all high risk children, (at the expense of the parent or guardian), due to the nature of a possible school injury, and to rule out diabetes. When Johnny was tested it was found he had pre-diabetes with chronically elevated sugar levels at age 10.

Johnny's mom also supported the idea that schools are fined for non-compliance with this new law. In her mind, this intervention with its incentives had possibly helped save her son's life! She found out how important proper incentives were for her family to continue to stay healthy. The state suggested that high risk schools must submit their plan within 180 days of designation as a BCEZ school in order to timely deal with the epidemic and to protect high risk children. Furthermore, School districts could be fined $1,000 a week, each week the plan is late.

Johnny's mother found out that all high risk children, at the end of the school year, must enroll in beta cell protection and a weight reduction training course, with their physician's approval, during the summer break. For those families who could not afford to pay for their child, or in the event the child could not participate in a certified program, the family must arrange for a volunteer to conduct similar training for them at home. Johnny would be expected to prepare a brief report over summer break regarding his understanding of the health and financial consequences of being overweight, and guess who agreed to help him write it? You guessed it--his biggest supporters: his parents.

Compliance is King

Fortunately for Johnny, the parents in his state read what happened in other states that had similar problems. What they found out was that the states that were successful needed to have some strong enforcement rules in place (similar to drunken driving offenders) so that the parents and schools would follow through on their part of the solution. Examples of this process are suggested in Chapter 1 Appendix 7.

The second aftershock: If the parents did not follow through with helping their high risk child, the state could impose a 1% garnishment of wages and salary (yes, this was drastic). This was levied on parents/guardians of high risk children that did not complete the high risk education after 2 years or more (garnishment ended once the education was completed). The states that had this rule in place had a 95% participation rate. The states that did not have this rule had a much lower participation rate. The successful states had mandatory PE instruction of children for 60 minutes a day by a certified trainer, educator, or volunteer. Even high risk college students over 18, based on their Body Mass Index (BMI) or belly button waist circumference measurement, completed an additional .5 credit hour per college year devoted to proper nutrition, as well as an additional .5 credit hour of physical education.

Since it was recognized by the parents that the epidemic was costing everyone a considerable amount of money, successful states implemented incentives to change the situation in BCEZ's. (See Chapter 1 Appendix Tables 8-9). They had mobile phone company incentives that included a reduced tax rate for every phone that downloaded a free, culturally appropriate, beta cell education application. If activated by an owner with a billing address in the epidemic zone, the phone owner obtained a discount on their next phone bill. These programs were highly successful in getting the word out about how to stop the epidemic.

The aftershocks keep rolling in: States also implemented BCEZ fast food incentives. In order to renew their food licenses, BCEZ fast food establishments distributed information about the economic impact of diabetes on children and the importance of beta cell health. All dessert menu items for all fast food category restaurants had a 20% consumption tax applied to support beta cell safety education in the state. BCEZ real estate incentives included higher property tax rates for fast food establishments. Taxes were automatically repealed once substantial changes were made to menus, as determined by the State Health Department.

Strikingly, real estate full-disclosures included the fact that the property being purchased was in a high risk epidemic zone that was potentially dangerous for children. As a result everyone owning real estate in the BCEZ zone became motivated to do something about the problem. Property taxes were lowered on all new property in the epidemic zone that created greater and safer access to physical activity areas for children and healthcare facilities for their families. Rates were also lowered for all new restaurants offering primarily a "kids health-friendly menu", as determined by the State Health Department.

Finally, as can be found in Chapter 1 Appendix Table 11, Johnny's state implemented insurance reform to help fight the epidemic. When Johnny's dad went to enroll in his employer's health insurance, he was notified of some substantial new changes. Insurance carriers were now allowed to charge higher premiums, deductibles, and copayments of at least a 10-20% differential for all adults and their adult dependents whose weight indicated they were involved in high risk eating behaviors. Due to the size of the epidemic, state insurance commissioners and health officials identified excessive over weight/obese adults and children as a preventable condition that needed immediate attention. State health officials considered obesity-related health costs as a primary factor in future state medical liability. The state felt the best way to handle the situation was to involve the employers in the state.

Johnny's dad's employer notified his dad that all employees and their adult dependents needed to complete a medical physical that confidentially reported their weight and BMI. His employer said that next year's insurance rates would definitely be going up for those employees and their adult dependents who were not in a healthy weight category, and who were smokers. This came as a shock to him, not so much the smoking idea, because he knew what smoking could do to his lungs. But, the weight criteria were shocking because he knew that he and Johnny's mom had a few pounds to lose before the next 12 months were up. The employer provided support counseling and web references on this important issue – an abbreviated list can be found in Appendix Table 10.

Space will not allow for a discussion of the myriad of additional incentives that can be introduced into our culture which can easily drive us away from the costly results of diabetes in our children. The time for plain talk is now, because type 2 diabetes in children is completely preventable and is at the level of epidemic proportions in our culture. There are simple solutions, including financial incentives that may work to curb this growing health problem. This book is dedicated to exploring those solutions and examining the financial impact of the loss of beta cells within the context of the responsibilities of government, families, physicians, and employers. First, do me a favor; just this one simple thing. Have a conversation in your family using the simple ideas presented below.

Chapter 1
Table 4
Fight diabetes and beta cell burnout as a family

1. We budget time and money to see a health professional annually because it saves us time and money and helps to insure our economic success.
2. We teach our child, our extended family, and our friends the vital importance of the pancreas' beta cells in keeping us healthy and productive.
3. We have economic incentives in our home that help children and adults to understand the financial benefit of eating wisely, including the benefits of greater financial freedom. We make it easy for all family

members to make correct choices and develop good habits by implementing economic consequences for our choices.

4. We work to obtain our personal healthy weight. We share with everyone that if you are young now, and are diagnosed with diabetes later on in life, the cost to you will be $500,000.

5. While being very economical, we create a healthy food environment at home, at school, and at work, based on the best elements of our traditional food culture

6. We abandon the unhealthy traditional foods, even if they are part of our ethnic heritage. Overeating high fat foods can bankrupt our children, their children, and our whole family.

7. We reduce our dependency on fast food because it is proven to be less than the best nutrition. If we eat too much fast food, it may cause us to grow poor and fat over time.

8. We participate in physical activity with our family for one hour a day. We know that active people are more successful and earn more money. Activity will keep our heart and lungs healthy. This is just what the heart doctor ordered!

9. We budget time and money to visit a healthcare professional immediately if we observe any signs of an food disorders in a family member including binge eating, purging, overeating, or excessive weight gain. Getting help earlier for these problems, rather than later may save our lives.

10. We remember that our beta cells produce insulin which is necessary for our bodies' energy. Without energy, we

cannot earn money and we will die prematurely. Beta cells are immensely important to our long-term health and financial security.

Chapter One Conclusions

I am pleased to announce that Johnny and his family are doing fabulously well. They eat healthily and exercise regularly. It took a combination of incentives at home, at school, and at work to get them on this path, but it worked. The family understands that their environment can overwhelm their self-control. They need to protect their family by changing their environment with the help of incentives.

I am convinced that every child and adult must know about the power of insulin and the exceeding importance of protecting the pancreas beta cells that produce it. Let us teach our young children the critical importance of preserving this vital organ in the same way we teach them to protect their teeth from cavities and avoid lung cancer by not smoking. Few, if any, children, let alone their parents, understand the necessity of protecting their pancreas' beta cells. It is time to enlist our free enterprise machine, both the public and private sectors, to foster solutions and incentives in the fight against beta cell burnout.

Johnny and his parents' journey can be a real story, a real success story. Remember that no amount of education or government initiatives to date have stemmed the obesity tide. We are all enlisted to fight this at the ground level, with our children close at hand. We can call on our schools, state and federal officials to help direct incentives that can impact this epidemic. As you will read throughout the remainder of this book, there are numerous ways to attack the problem that cost little or no money. The only cost is our pride, our traditions, and our way of thinking. I am convinced that we can shape a healthy future, but it will require a new way of thinking, and it will require new incentives to be successful. Read on for more economic tactics to fight against the loss of our beta cells. I am a big believer that solutions can be found for all of our problems by working first and foremost in our families. So, let us examine how any typical family can take on the battle for the life and the health of their beta cells.

Chapter 1
Appendix

Nutritional and Activity Based Economic Motivations for
Children

Disclaimer: All children who are severely overweight
are at risk for developing diabetes and need to promptly
visit a medical provider. Professional treatment plans need
to be closely followed. The following is not a treatment
plan.

- Many young women have eating disorders. Please be
  extremely cautious and observant in dealing with issues
  of weight management;
- If your healthcare professional considers that your child
  is at risk for developing diabetes, take their
  recommendations seriously and follow them closely.
  Take action on behalf of your child.
- If you, your spouse, or the child's guardians are at risk
  for developing diabetes, seek medical attention. Follow
  your treatment plan carefully, and implement your own
  economic motivators.

Chapter 1
Appendix Table 1
American Dietetic Association

Consider what the American Dietetic Association report as the elements of successful nutrition incentives at: http://www.hc-sc.gc.ca/fn-an/label-etiquet/nutrition/educat/strat_framework_entire-cadre_strat_entier-04-eng.php.

Chapter 1
Appendix Table 1 continued
Keys to Successful Nutrition Education
American Dietetic Association
Partial summary of best practice principles

- Consumer-driven nutrition education programs developed on the basis of the needs, behaviors, motivations and desires of target audiences;
- A focus on influencing the consumer, *going beyond merely providing information and incorporating methods for actually creating behavior change to bridge the gap between consumers' awareness of nutrition and their actual practices* **[emphasis added]**; and
- Delivering the information in a form a consumer can actually use to improve their diet;
- Include active involvement of both the individual and the community;
- Use of multiple, reinforcing, interactive channels of communication;

(Source: see above link)

Economic ramifications may be important to help all of us, especially our children, sustain healthy nutrition and exercise habits. For any child who is at risk for losing their beta cell function, special attention may be required. Not all incentives may be appropriate to our own family's or child's circumstances. Here are some ground rules to consider.

Chapter 1
Appendix Table2
Ground Rules for Assisting Children

- Love your child unconditionally, in every circumstance.
- Lead by example. Be authoritative, not authoritarian. Use these economic motivations in a supportive fashion.
- Set reasonable individual goals for proper nutrition and exercise (follow your healthcare professional recommendations).
- Ensure the home environment is super supportive of proper nutrition and exercise, and that all family members are role models to one another.
- Use economic motivation along with education to protect your child from high risk behavior.
- Collaborate with your child to engage the economics of motivation, appropriate to their age, by connecting high risk behaviors with an economic consequence.

Now that we have established the ground rules of seeing a professional first if you or your child is in need of medical care, and that these strategies are only suggestions for discussion, we can move on to the next step in the process of finding solutions to the epidemic of diabetes.

The assertion is that there are economic consequences to behavior. To support you and your child's goals direct your child's attention to the following activity.

Chapter 1

Appendix Table 3

Economic Incentives for Children to Encourage Proper Nutrition and Exercise at Home

Instructions for parents with children at high risk for developing diabetes:

1. Please note, these are examples of activities that reinforce economic consequences for health choices.
2. Select items based on your perceived importance to your child.
3. Gain agreement, create a contract. As a reference please visit http://www.rewardingkids.com/tools-to-change-behavior/behavior-contract/.
4. Praise your child for any and all efforts made to become more physically fit.
5. Emphasize the tremendous economic value of being fit and avoiding health problems.
6. Reinforce the principle that eating well and exercising are rewarding. Both can help you earn more money, as well as more time to do the things you want to do.
7. Together with your children, pick a couple of items from below and combine them with health behaviors. For instance, if your child eats more green vegetables and less sweets they can have more or less:

- Allowance
- Vacation time budgeted for their interests
- Phone use
- Friend time
- Computer use
- Entertainment funds for movies, music, etc.
- Clothing allowance
- Hobbies
- TV time
- Gas money (walk or ride to school)
- Car money
- Tuition
- Room and board
- More/less of anything of economic value the child suggests will motivate them

Try the same with activity levels. Your children can earn more or less of these items if they are more active in walking, sports, chores or any other form of physical exercise. Be sure to track the results, be generous and make the reward meaningful. Above all make sure that your love for your child transcends this process.

This process is important and has real meaning for their lives. As you see improvements in their healthy choices, such as more activity and more vegetables being eaten, make sure you praise them. Also, do not forget the consequences. If the agreed upon goals are not met, make sure you hold them accountable to a loss of something that is meaningful to them. The behavioral scientist may suggest that these items may be earned initially, but they are theirs to lose. In other words, give the allowance automatically at the beginning of the week, but remind them that there will be no allowance next week if they do not follow through.

Chapter 1
Appendix Table 4
Economic Incentives for Children to Encourage Proper Nutrition and Exercise at School

New ideas are necessary to stimulate the discussion around solutions to the diabetes epidemic. To be sure, these next possible solutions are a different and unique way to approach the problem, and are as yet unproven. What _is_ proven is that the majority of us are motivated to some degree _economically,_ and therefore it is ethically appropriate to examine our problem in the light of monetary consequences.

Nutrition and Exercise at School
Primary Incentives in a School Environment:
A brief, mandatory questionnaire, for all students, administered to determine students' understanding of:
• The financial implications of overeating
• Beta cell health
• Nutrition, exercise
• Risk of diabetes

General instructions for students, parents, teachers and volunteers:
1. Please remember this type of intervention may be necessary to help stop the diabetes epidemic.

2. Recognize that all of us, and especially children, are hypersensitive about our appearance, especially our weight.
3. Keep all incentives economic in nature, otherwise this becomes an exercise in general education which, to date, has not been proven very effective.

Specific Instructions for Student Questionnaire

1. Required by all students 3rd grade through college, with the oversight of a parent and guardian where appropriate.
2. Children must submit the completed questionnaire within 90 days to their home room teacher.
3. Distributed by and approved by the school. Conducted either online, at school, by mobile phone, by land line, by text message, by a class volunteer, by fax, during school, by PTA, or by any other method approved by the school district.

Basic Economic Incentive Suggestion

Nutrition and physical fitness *questionnaire*

- Questionnaire content: age appropriate nutrition and activity education.
- Incentives:
  - School collects a $5.00 fee to administer this education.
  - A child's guardian is fined $30 dollars a month up to $200 dollars in any given school year, if the questionnaire is not completed within the first 60 days of school attendance.
  - Added Incentive:
  - Qualifies children for school lunch program.

- o Random drawing from submitted questionnaires so individual students can win the chance to help select special items from the pre-approved menu.
- Content
  - o Annual, mandatory completion of nutritional education in English and native tongue.
  - o Ongoing mandatory monthly curriculum content includes, nutrition, diet, exercise education, and beta cell importance.

Chapter 1

Appendix Table 5

Substantial Economic Incentives Suggestions for Schools to Consider

(Example of a substantial economic incentive: Drunk drivers are required to enroll in treatment programs, at their own expense.)

Each student in the state is weighed (all weight data is deleted except for those children at severe risk. Average weight per grade/gender/age is calculated)

- Each adult student must supply their Body Mass Index (BMI) (again, all weight data is deleted except for those children at severe risk).
- Automatic enrollment in nutrition, beta cell protection and activity education for high risk children and their parent/ guardians.
- High risk criteria are determined by State Health Department Standards .

- All costs for the education of these children and adults are borne by the high risk adult student, or in the case of high risk minors, their respective parent or guardian.
- Payment penalties up to $200 dollars for failure to complete the prescribed education within 60 days.
- Additional automatic enrollment of high risk children and their parents in 6 volunteer, (peer-to-peer) lead classes where feasible.

Educational Classes

1. #1 class taught by a type 1 diabetic patient. Subject: Living with Diabetes.
2. #2 in 5 parts: Video education documenting the medical and economic impact of type 2 diabetes:
   A) Risk of and economic burden of stroke
   B) Risk of and economic burden of amputation
   C) Risk of and economic burden of heart attack
   D) Risk of and economic burden of kidney failure
   E) Risk of and economic burden of blindness

Chapter 1

Appendix Table 6

Creating Epidemic Zones (EZ):

Economic leverage is created by leveraging weight statistics

Instructions:

1. To protect children: States, counties, cities, or communities create epidemic zones (EZ), or beta cell endangerment zones BCEZ.

2. EZ are identified where the population of children at risk is highest, based on weight statistics.

3. Statistics are blinded for each students except for those who are at high risk.

4. Statistics are compiled by the state to calculate averages to assess the relative risks of diabetes and obesity.

5. Each school records and submits the number of children at risk for diabetic or obesity.

6. Each EZ school submits a parent approved plan to assist all children attending to understand the importance both economically and medically of staying physically fit.

7. Physical examinations are automatically scheduled for all high risk children, at the expense of the parent or guardian, due to nature of possible injury at school, and to rule out type 2 diabetes.

8. Schools are fined for non-compliance.

9. EZ information is announced publically:
   a. Percentages of at risk children published.
   b. Parents of students attending schools in the EZ zone are notified in writing, via normal school channels, 3 times a year.

Incentives

- High risk schools must submit their plan to deal with epidemic and to assist high risk children within 180 days of designation as an EZ school.
    - o School districts are fined $1,000 a week, each week the plan is late.
    - o Included in the plan are financial incentives for parents.
- All high risk children, at the end of the school year:
    - o Enroll in beta cell protection, weight reduction training course (with their physician's approval, during the summer break.
        - The cost of completion is responsibility of the family.
            - Expectation that the child earns the money through summer employment.
        - Certified when completed
            - Those families who cannot afford to pay for their child, or, in the event the child cannot participate in a certified program, the family arranges for a volunteer to conduct similar training for them at home.
    - o Prepare a brief report over summer break regarding their understanding of the medical and economic consequences of the disease.

Chapter 1

Appendix Table 7

Culturally Significant Economic Incentives

Suggestions to Protect and Support our Children at Risk

Instructions:

1. The following suggestions may seem extreme and challenging to our sense of individual freedom. The suggestions are offered, nonetheless, in an ethical manner, in response to creating the necessary incentives to fight the spread of the diabetes epidemic.

2. In some cases these suggestions require legislation and union negotiations.

Incentives (drastic):

- 1% garnishment of wages and salary.
- Applied to parents/guardians of high risk children that remain in the high risk category for 2 years or more.
- This garnishment is held as a health savings account and is accessed to pay for health related expenses including for the medical education and treatment of their child.
- Mandatory PE instruction of children for 60 minutes a day, by a certified trainer/educator/volunteer.
- Parent Teacher Association charter incentive:
- Charter to include a requirement to have activities sponsoring proper nutritional and exercise, including beta cell education.
- EZ school employment contracts for new teachers, and new administrators, by virtue of their position as a role model for children:

- Applicants are ineligible for employment if they are in a high risk health category including obesity and smoking.
- Applicants must qualify by simply measuring waist circumference (not waist size) based the world wide evidence of risk for diabetes, as published in the national guidelines published by the American Diabetes. Association and the American Heart Association.
- High risk college students over 18, based on their BMI, or waist circumference:
  o Must complete an additional 1 credit hour per year devoted to proper nutrition, exercise, with curriculum that:
    - Discusses the importance of protecting beta cell function.
    - Offers suggestions on how to avoid the economic and medical consequences of type 2 diabetes, and other diseases caused by chronic overeating.
  o High risk students complete an additional 2 credit hours of P.E. as a requirement for graduating.

Chapter 1

Appendix Table 8

<u>Additional High Impact Economic Incentives Suggestion to</u>

<u>help stop the Spread of Diabetes</u>

- Epidemic Zone (EZ) Mobile Phone Carrier Incentives
  - o Phone numbers registered on social media sites to minors with Area codes that are within EZ.
    - Include public service announcements pop ups.
    - Advises minors of the risk of chronic overeating.
    - Recommend children struggling with eating disorders see a medical professional to discuss their problem with a school counselor, parent or guardian and/ or any health professional.
  - o Cell phone carriers download free culturally appropriate, child safe, beta cell education applications. If activated by an owner with a billing address in the epidemic zone, the phone owner can obtain a discount on their next phone bill.
- EZ Fast Food Restaurant Incentives:
  - o EZ Fast food establishments to distribute information on the <u>economic impact</u> of diabetes on children, and the importance of beta cells.

- o All dessert menu items for all fast food category restaurants have a 20% consumption tax applied to support beta cell safety education.
- EZ Real Estate Incentives
    - o Higher property tax rates for fast food establishments. Taxes are repealed once substantial changes are made to menus, as determined by the State Health Department.
    - o Real estate disclosures must include the fact that the property being purchased is in a high risk epidemic zone that is potentially dangerous for children.
    - o Property taxes are lowered on all new property in the epidemic zone that creates greater and safer access to physical activity areas for children and healthcare facilities for their families.
    - o Property taxes are lowered on all new restaurants offering primarily a kids health friendly menu as determined by the State Health Department.
    - o Property taxes are decreased for activity centers designed for children as the primary clientele (e.g. gyms).
- State Constitutional Budgetary Amendments:
    - o Require infrastructure modifications in epidemic zones to allow greater access to safe recreation for children.
- Food:
    - o EZ sugared beverages sales have a 50% sales tax levied.

o Computer/video game manufactures that produce games for children that encourage physical activity receive tax incentives.

Chapter 1
Appendix Table 9
Additional School Incentives

- Approved school lunch menu meet nutritional standards and be culturally appropriate, or fines may be imposed.
- In schools with the highest risk and rate of diabetes, school lunch menus are monitored by the state government.

Chapter 1
Appendix Table 10
Additional Web Sites

For more information on specific resources for children with diabetes visit these web sites:

- American Diabetes Association - www.diabetes.org
- Juvenile Diabetes Research Foundation - www.jdrf.org/
- Centers for Disease Control - www.cdc.gov/diabetes/projects/diab_children.htm
- Your state's health department

Chapter 1

Appendix Table 11

State Insurance Reform to Protect and Support Children
from Beta Cell Loss

Insurance:

- All healthcare insurance carriers can charge higher premiums, deductibles, and copayments of at least a 10-20% differential for all adults and their adult dependents whose weight indicate they are at high risk <u>for preventable</u> obesity.
    - State insurance commission identifies excessive over weight/obese children as engaged in high risk behavior due to the probability of developing diabetes and the loss of beta cell function.
    - Additional health insurance for high risk children is made available for purchase by the parent or guardian of high risk children.
    - Obesity in the vast majority of cases is preventable, which empowers the State insurance commission to develop policies that allow for preventative economic incentives to become part of all employer health benefit designs.

Note: See Medicaid and Medicare chapters for information on how incentives can reform Medicaid and Medicare

Chapter 1
Reference List

Oral Diabetes Medications. Brunilda Nazario. WebMD, LLC., 2011.

Butler, Alexandra E., et al. "Cell Deficit and Increased Cell Apoptosis in Humans With type 2 Diabetes." Diabetes 52.1 (2003): 102-10.

CDC Division of Media Relations. Number of Americans with Diabetes Projected to Double or Triple by 2050. 2010.

Centers for Disease Control and Prevention. National diabetes fact sheet: general information and national estimates on diabetes in the United States, 2007.U.S. Department of Health and Human Services, Centers for Disease Control and Prevention, 2008, 2011.

National diabetes fact sheet: national estimates and general information on diabetes and prediabetes in the United States, 2011. U.S. Department of Health and Human Services, Centers for Disease Control and Prevention, 2011, 2011.

U.S. Obesity Trends.Centers for Disease Control and Prevention, 2011.

Rabin, Roni Caryn. "Prognosis: Numbers Rise in a Diabetes Forecast." The New York Times 30 Nov. 2009.

Rubenstein, Ed. "The Economics of Crime." IMPRIMIS Because Ideas Have Consequences (1995).

U.S.Department of Health and Human Services. Yesterday, Today, and Tomorrow: NIH Research Timelines. 2011.

Zhuo, X. Estimated Lifetime Cost for Diabetes Higher for Male Patients. 2011.

$$\Sigma$$

CHAPTER 2

Families in Jeopardy

<u>The most educated parents in the world are also the heaviest</u>

Here are some astounding economic facts. American parents living in arguably the most developed country in the world, are losing their beta cell function at 2.5 times the rate of parents living in a "developing" country like China. American parents spend 50 times more on diabetes expenditures than Latin and South American countries. (IDF Diabetes Atlas 5th Edition) If parents are financially fortunate enough to have insurance, they are generally better educated, and have a higher risk for developing diabetes. Compounding this phenomenon is the fact that poor parents in wealthy countries eat more of what is bad for them (i.e. high sugar and high saturated fat food).

Our research effort is not helping us avoid obesity. We spend almost all of our research and education dollars (author estimated at 100 to 1) learning about and teaching nutrition and exercise, while little or no money is spent on

research to determine economic forces that will keep us from eating too much. Recently, D.A. Booth noted in the journal *Appetite*:

> ...no research has been funded into the public's descriptions of feasible changes that cause a step down in weight, let alone into the environmental conditions for individuals' maintenance of those changes. As a result, public health policies on obesity lack scientific basis; (Booth DA 210-21)

Although we do not have good research on how to motivate us to protect our beta cells, we have tremendous research on the risks and costs associated with diabetes.

Chapter 2

Table 1

Estimated Lifetime Risk of Developing Diabetes for Individuals Born in the United States in 2000

Percent Risk

- Men 32%
    - White 28%
    - Black 40%
    - Hispanic 45%

- Women 38%
    - White 30%
    - Black 49%
    - Hispanic 52%

(Narayan et al, JAMA, 2003)

To understand how to motivate families to fight this epidemic we need to understand economic motivations that directly apply to families that are at high risk. According to recent American Diabetes Association (ADA) and the National Institutes of Health (NIH) statistics, if we have diabetes, we will spend between 2,000 and 11,000 dollars a year on expenses-related medical costs (or 2-6 times higher than for others using medical services in a given year).(American Diabetes Association) Take a point in between, $6,000, to highlight our discussion. Or, compare this $6,000 figure to the following:

- The average costs of owning and operating a car is $8,000
- The average cost of college tuition per year is $7,500
- The median US household income is $50,000

The economic consequences created by the loss of our beta cells can dramatically worsen an average family's financial situation. Based on the above $6,000 figure, a median income family would spend approximately 10% of their income on diabetes related expenses. This may cause a family to forfeit economic essentials such as a college education or reliable transportation.

It may be appropriate to take a longer term financial perspective in order to see the direct costs that affect a bread winner. Again, according to ADA statistics, if diabetes strikes you between the ages of 18 and 34, your loss of earnings (primarily due to an early death) will be over $500,000. (American Diabetes Association 596-615) This is almost equivalent to what a 30 year old needs to save, if they hope to retire at a median US income of $50,000 a year.

If we are like most of the folks that will become diagnosed with diabetes in our 40's and 50's, we can expect to lose, on average, between $400,000 and $700,000 dollars in lifetime earnings. (American Diabetes Association 596-615) This is ten times more than the average person saves for retirement. To protect our loved ones from our overeating and lack of activity, we need to double the amount of contributions we are putting into retirement, because we can count on our earning potential being substantially reduced.

There may be some who doubt these financial statistics. Consider another point of view. At age 50, men with diabetes will lose almost two weeks' worth of pay, or roughly $2,000 a year, primarily by utilizing health resources. Compared to a healthy male, on average a 50 year old man with a substantial loss of beta cell function will annually:

1. Spend more time in the hospital
2. Spend more days in the emergency room
3. Spend more days visiting their health provider
(American Diabetes Association 596-615)

These two weeks of pay, lost to medical costs, could add up to a household's entire vacation time, or an entire budget for their children's extracurricular school activities. Furthermore, the economist might point out that to motivate financial behavior there needs to be a fair exchange of values. Remember, economic principles are not in and of themselves mean-spirited, but they can represent reality. What then is the fair exchange of value of preventing diabetes in our households? Examples from successfully motivated families may be conversations like:

1. College contract discussion: Our maintenance of a healthy weight (not too heavy or too thin) is worth, on average $6,000 to our family. Please choose your food and exercise wisely. Our first (or next semester) college fund may be in jeopardy otherwise.

2. Car contract discussion: Our maintenance of a healthy weight (not too heavy or too thin) is vitally important to our financial health. In fact, it is probably worth $6,000 to our family's annual budget, <u>or $500 a month</u>. Please choose your food and exercise wisely. Your auto allowance may be in jeopardy otherwise.

3. Doubling retirement contributions, a discussion with a spouse: Let's consult our retirement expert. Our retirement earning potential may be severely restricted if we chronically overeat. If we continue to do so, <u>we may need to double our monthly contributions</u> in order retire as planned!

Now for a longer, more sobering statistic, consider an end-of-life common occurrence.

<u>Long Term Care Costs</u>

- 1 in 3 seniors (65 and older) will be admitted to nursing homes (Disturbing Statistics about Long Term Care in the US)
- 24% of all nursing home patients are estimated to have diabetes (Centers for Disease Control and Prevention)
- The average annual cost of stay in a nursing home is $70,000- $80,000
- The average length of stay is 2.5 years and approximately $200,000 (Centers for Disease Control and Prevention)

- The median single family home sold for less than $200,000 in 2010 (www. Realtor.org)

This means that if our primary asset in life is a home that we proudly own outright, the government will take possession of it at the end of our life, in order to cover the cost of our diabetes care in a nursing home. As senior citizens, we will have a substantial risk of entering a nursing home at the end of our lives. If we do not have the assets to cover the cost of care, we may need to consider the substantial financial impact. The conversation might look something like this:

"My dear family, we have all worked hard to pay for and maintain this home over our lifetime. We need to consider that if we endanger our health through our poor eating habits and poor exercise habits, we will not be able to keep our home in our family. We will need to cede our home to the federal government to help cover the cost of our medical care."

This is a harsh reality, clearly a cause for serious contemplation as we plan for our financial futures. Perhaps we should consider purchasing additional insurance to cover the cost of a nursing home stay. Here is an estimated premium for nursing home insurance:

- 55 year old in good health, without diabetes – approx. $1800 – or roughly $140 a month (Long-Term Care Insurance)
- 55 year old with diabetes – may not be offered by any insurance company

A wise retirement advisor would suggest that in order to protect our assets (from our over-eating), we need to begin budgeting $140 a month if we are in mid-life. If we purchase this long-term healthcare insurance later in life, we may need to budget $500 dollars or more in our monthly insurance budget. Less than 1 in 10 seniors have insurance to cover nursing home costs. (Day)

No wonder the government can request our assets to cover the cost of our care. The economist would ask this question: why shouldn't the government take our assets earlier in our lives if we willingly participate in high risk behaviors? As we will see in later chapters, the government may need to do so, or risk the bankruptcy of Medicare and Medicaid.

What are your Risks?

Examining our personal risks may lead us to implement positive family incentives to help the family avoid preventable adverse economic outcome. Let us begin with something that many families dream of—owning a Cadillac. To examine how your family can afford buying a Cadillac, take this little quiz on the next page.

Chapter 2

Table 2

Economic Motivators for Families

How to Buy Our First Cadillac

Instructions: Please place an X under the column that applies. X = 1 point

	Heavy?	Stroke, Heart, Kidneys?
Mother:		
Father:		
Spouse:		
A Sibling:		
Best Friend:		
First Child:		
Total Points:	_____ +	_____ = Total points (12 possible)

Interpreting your family's risk for significant economic impact of the loss of beta cell function:

If we are overweight and scored an 8 or higher, our family is <u>at high risk</u> and needs to see a healthcare professional. If we are severely overweight, our children have a 50% chance of being obese. That risk rises to 80% if both parents are severely over weight (obese). (Facts for Families: Obesity in Children and teens)

If a child is heavy by age 13, there is an 80% chance they are at high risk for beta cell burnout as an adult. If we are severely obese, we have a high chance of losing our beta cells and passing on a poor nutritional environment to our children. (Mokdad et al. 76-79) If we are related to, or are close friends with, or are currently ourselves overweight, we may need to budget for additional healthcare costs.

The loss of beta cells now produces a hidden tax of $700 for every American citizen, or for a family of four, $2800 a year ($233 month). (Dall et al. 297-303) On top of that, even if no family member is currently diagnosed with diabetes, a family of four needs to budget substantially for direct medical costs associated with pre-diabetes (i.e. being moderately overweight). The amount recently calculated is $443 per pre-diabetic person, per year, or $1772 per family of four per year, ($148 per month). Including taxes paid, and direct medical costs incurred, a family of four needs to budget $381 per month for the care related to the loss of beta cells. <u>Approximately 90% or $342 of this cost is avoidable</u>. Let's put all of this into a motivating economic incentive. The cost to lease a new Cadillac is, as advertised at the time of this writing,

<u>$399 a month</u>

<u>Bottom line</u>: By saving our beta cells a family of four can lease a new Cadillac.

There is even more shocking news than if our close friends can see us driving up in our brand new Cadillac. Our friendships could be preventing us from buying the Cadillac. How do we know that, and why are friends listed in the risk table above? Because recent evidence suggests that not only is there a cost to what we and our families are doing to our beta cells, but there is also a cost to what friendships we enjoy. We see this in the way that body fat may follow us into our close friendships.

Chapter 2
Table 3
Impact of Friends

Quotes from an article published in the *New England Journal of Medicine*. (Statistical methodologies involved in this study are under debate)

"The Spread of Obesity in a Large Social Network over 32 Years" (Christakis and Fowler 370-79)

Broad study findings are directly quoted:

- A person's chances of becoming obese increased by 57% if he or she had a friend who became obese.
- The closeness of friendship is relevant to the spread of obesity.
- Persons in closer, mutual friendships have more of an effect on each other than persons in other types of friendships.

Compare this to:

- ...if one sibling became obese, the chance that the other would become obese increased by 40%
- If one spouse became obese, the likelihood that the other spouse would become obese increased by 37%

We have established that inordinate weight gain puts our beta cells at risk. Compare the impact of one close friend on your finances. Is our closest friend slender, overweight or obese? Are we slender, overweight, or over-eating? What financial impact are we having on our friends and their families? And, if you are a mother, you may be especially interested with the economic impact of overeating.

Chapter 2

Table 4

A Heavy Burden: The Individual Costs of Being
Overweight and Obese in the United States (Dor et al. 1-27)

The overall, tangible, annual costs* of being obese are:

- $4,879 for an obese woman [$407 a month, ~ $14 dollars a day]
- $2,646 for an obese man [$220 a month, ~$7 a dollars a day]
- $534 for an overweight woman [$ 45 month, ~ $ 1.5 dollars a day]
- $432 for an overweight man [$36month, ~ $1.2 a dollars a day]

*Most of these costs are medically driven.

For the purposes of our discussion, we will assume the mother is obese and the father is overweight. This produces an annual burden on the family of approximately $450 a month or $15 dollars a day; a magical number. (National Occupational Employment and Wage Estimates) The median hourly wage in America is between $15 and $16 dollars a day. So, in our example, Dad or Mom is working on average, an hour extra every day, of every year, for the rest of our lives, just to afford to be heavy.

We are going to put that extra hour back into our lives, and $15 back into our pockets with the following incentives. As an at-risk family, stop what you are doing and consider doing this—it works.

Family Incentives

To stop the painful loss of this money and immediately begin to improve our health, we must feel the financial pain of our eating choices every day. Behavioral scientists tell us the fear of loss is greater than the hope to gain. And, to date, small amounts of money, won or rewarded for weight loss, has had only moderate success in changing behavior.

Motivational theory may also teach us that rewards and punishments need to be immediate, constant and consistent with the size of the problem. In theory, if we follow economic principles outlined above, <u>we must put at financial risk the cost of our behavior</u>. This equates on average to: $450 dollars a month, or $15 a day, or at least 10% of our income.

What does it mean to put our own money at risk? In principle, to ensure we are adequately motivated, we must lose the money. We lose the money, for example, if and only if, we fail to lose weight and protect our beta cells. For the family incentive to work, it must have a direct consequence that results in a real financial loss. The deducted money must be considered lost. Remember, the fear of loss is greater than hope to gain. Fear of really losing ten percent of your income, the amount we lose if we remain at an unhealthy weight, is the root solution for our financial motivation to regain our health.

In reality, this is not as easy as it sounds. We must take the money we would spend on excess medical costs, clothing, food, gasoline, etc., and put it at risk! What person in their right mind would ever do this? Answer: Those, like us, that know **if it is not done, IT IS LOST FOR SURE!** We cannot beat the healthcare costs of weight gain—it is physically and financially impossible. That course is proven. So, review this family plan that can help us change our environment and put strong incentives into our daily routine that can help us change. The following plan is not original to the author*.

Chapter 2

Table 5

Plan A: The Super Successful, Fear of Loss, Family
Financial Plan

Or, simply said: $100 per pound plan, guaranteed to work or your money lost!

1. See a physician, buy a scale, and seek advice on proper nutrition and exercise.
2. Create and stick to a budget.
3. Find an anti-charity (an organization that everyone in the family despises).
4. Goals: establish, with your physician's approval, a goal to lose one pound a week. This goal is worth approximately:
   a. $15 a day, as in our example family above
   b. $100 a week
   c. $100 a pound
5. Write a check out to the anti-charity for $450 or 10% of your monthly income. Put it in an envelope that is preaddressed and stamped. Tape it to your mirror.
6. At the close of each month, weigh your overweight participating family members.
7. If participants lose 4 pounds during the month, do not mail the check.

8. If participants do not lose 4 pounds during the month, mail the check. If you do not have the willpower to do so, ask a friend, guardian, or spouse to mail it for you.

9. Continue until all family members are at their normal weight.

*Fortunately, there are a few ingenious websites, designed to help us implement this plan. You can actually set up an account that allows you to put your money at risk. If the envelope trick does not work for you, and a guardian is not available, check out these sites for added reinforcement. They may give you the added edge you need to meet your healthy weight goals: *www.stickk.com; and *www.healthywage.com.

If your family does not have access to a banking relationship, open a piggy-bank instead. Still select a guardian, and every week put a $100 dollars or 10% of your income into an envelope, and slip it into the piggy bank that is protected by the guardian. Follow the rest of the plan as outlined, especially the part of having the guardian give the money to an organization who opposes your values. Now you have the BIG incentive to change.

If we cannot stomach the pain of putting at risk $450 or 10% of our budget, here is another option for us:

Chapter 2
Table 6
The EAC out Plan

This program is guaranteed to work or your money lost!

The idea of the EAC out Plan: Put your budget, (E) for entertainment, (A) for alcohol, and (C) for cigarettes at risk as incentive to save your family's beta cells.

The EAC out Plan

The average American family (2.5 persons) spends the following on entertainment, alcohol and cigarettes:

- Entertainment (E): $ 2,700 a year or $225 a month, or $7 a day
- Alcohol (A): $450 a year, $38 a month, or ~$1 a day
- Cigarettes (C): $323 a year, $27 a month, or ~1 a day
- Total EAC expenditures: $3,473 a year, $290 round up to $300 a month, or ~ $9-10 a day
- Now compare:
  - Annual expenditures for food at home $3460
  - Annual expenditures for EAC items $3,470.
  - Notice that these two categories are virtually equal

An average family has between $200 a month (if we are a non-smoker non-drinker) and $300 a month (if we also smoke and drink) to help motivate the family to change. This is the EAC incentive. It is a strong enough incentive to keep the family healthy. The incentive is the equivalent of $6-$10 a day that can be put at risk to motivate change. This incentive does not, on average, affect our financial stability. To keep to our budget, we will need to cancel all forms of entertainment for us and our children.

This is a painful choice, but one that will quickly bring results. Why? We can earn all of the money back by losing 1 pound a month. Everyone can stay whole if the healthy eating and activity levels are followed. Yes there will be consternation, complaining, possibly even raised voices. Here is the conversation to have with your family.

"Dear family, we are at risk for losing our home in our old age. We are all at risk for killing off our beta cells too early. Currently we are at greater risk for blindness, kidney failure, stroke, amputation and injury. We are at risk for losing $400,000 in income by dying early or by putting our jobs on the line because we may not be as productive as others. We are in need of changing our behavior, our environment, and our incentives so we can stay healthy and protect our beta cells. The plan we are going to embrace will allow us to each lose a pound a week and avoid all of the problems we just mentioned. Can we all support this plan?"

As a family, follow the instructions above and write out a check, or put cash in an envelope addressed and stamped so it can be sent to an organization you are morally opposed to supporting. This becomes your hated anti-charity donation that you are loath to donate to, in the event your family goal is not met. The amount of the check needs to be $200-$300. Stop all entertainment for 90 days, if the goals are met, restore the E part of the EAC budget and live happily ever after.

Dianomics tells it like it is: The larger the potential monetary loss, the greater the chances for personal change. If we cannot find a piggy bank or a guardian to help us follow through on this plan, economists rightly assume we are not ready to change, and our family will pay on average $450 dollars a month for the rest of our time together to cover increased medical and other costs associated with poor nutritional choices. The physician we see will tell us that we will eventually also lose our beta cells and become a person with preventable diabetes.

We first and foremost work to give birth, protect, feed, and shelter our children and families. Incentives to change our habits must be strong enough to impact our ability to accomplish the purposes of this most important work.

Previously, we suggested, based on economics, that loss-aversion, or the fear-of loss-now, is greater than the hope-to-gain in the future. An important part of this theory of motivation is that the size of the <u>potential loss or gain must be substantial</u>. Do we have a scenario to support our premise of change motivation that includes a short term hope to gain emphasis? Yes indeed.

To see this scenario clearly, consider the impact of our everyday decisions and the financial impact on our personal and family life. Assume for the sake of this discussion, that we are endangering our beta cells and that our family is overweight or obese. Overweight is defined as at least 10% over a healthy weight, and obese is defined as 30% over our healthy weight. Taking the rough average we are overspending approximately 20% to feed ourselves if we are obese or overweight. <u>In food costs alone,</u> we have a hope to gain scenario of a least $1200 a year for an average family that is overweight. In other words, $100 a month for an average family for the rest of their time together is our hope to gain, provided that we eat less. Remember this $100 as we make the following comparisons. What can my family do with an additional $100 per month of disposable income? Put this $100 in an envelope and motivate yourself and your family with a positive incentive.

- 1 month saved buys a gym pass for 3-4 months
- 3 months saved buys a nice bicycle
- 6 months saved buys a laptop computer

- In six months, save enough for 2 Haitian children to attend school every day for a full year
- In one year, save enough to cover food costs for a college student
- In five years, save a reasonable down payment for a home

Here are some additional startling statistics that our friendly economists hope we understand. We can use them so we can better protect our families and support better economic alternatives. (Godsey)

http://kroger.staywellsolutionsonline.com/Library/Wellness

- (From the authors own calculation), one dollar buys approximately 300 calories, on average.
- American men, on average, consume 30% more calories than we need. That equates to 600 or more calories a day than is needed for good nutrition. Or, to further calculate, it equates to at least $2 a day, $60 dollars a month or $720 a year spent on wasted or excess food, for every American man.
- 90 million men waste, on average, $180,000,000 a day on food (Spraggins 1-19).

Now, you thought the women were going to get off the hook. However, economists are equal opportunity focused.

- If women eat out frequently, they likely consume an excess of 300 or more calories a day. In 6 weeks, they may actually put on a pound of weight compared to normal eaters. At this rate, they will be 8 pounds heavier in a year.
- In addition, this overeating is costing, at minimum, an extra $1 dollar a day, $30 a month and $365 dollars a

year. This covers the cost of a phone, or manicures/pedicures, or a 30 minute massage each month.

- If women eat out at fast food restaurants they eat more calories in fat and less of the good stuff, like fruits and vegetables. Bottom line: if we eat at fast food restaurants 5-6 times as week, we will be fatter than those who do not, <u>and we will be putting our beta cells at risk.</u> (Strong, Parks, and Anderson 1708-15),(Price and Taste Trump Nutrition When Americans Eat Out)

<u>Milk vs. Soda:</u>
- 4 cups of milk have 32 grams of protein, and can be purchased for one dollar.
- 1 can of soda has 0 nutritional value, and it too can be purchased for one dollar.

The economist would suggest a few very simple, yet immediately impactful changes to our home environment. These suggestions will save us $100 a month, and help us to not lose the $450 or 10% of our income we may need to put at risk each month to help us change.

<u>Suggestions</u>
1. Stop purchasing any foods that have no nutritional value. Added sugar calories, in any form, do not count as nutrition.
2. Ask ourselves this question before purchasing an item: "If I ate this three times a day, would it be bad for me?" If so do not buy it, or eat it, even if we are going to eat it only once a year!

3. Tell all of our friends and family what we are risking, and if appropriate, ask for their help and participation. Let's show them the money we have at risk!

4. Importantly, be an example of nutrition and exercise to your whole family.

   A California report found:

   - o Nearly half of adolescents (48 percent) whose parents drink soda every day, eat fast food at least once a day [which means these children are put at risk for losing their beta cells earlier]
   - o Every day, more than 2 million California adolescents (62 percent) drink soda (New Factor in Teen Obesity: Parents)

5. Please see Table 7 for statistics that put our eating habits into perspective: (Visual Economics, 2011, 22 /id)

Chapter 2

Table 7

Food Facts that matter for the average American Family (2.5 consumers)

- Food at home: 7% of household income or $3,465, per year
- Food away from home 5.4% household income or $2,668, per year
- Total food: 12.4% or $6,133, per year (rising steadily)
- Food costs per day, average $16.80 per family
- Food costs per person per day is $6.75
- Food costs per month, average $504 per family
- Average recommended calories per person, per day 2,000 (5,000 per average family)

- Average recommended calories per family per year (5,000 calories x 365 days) = 1,825,000 calories per year, per average family. Bet you didn't know that one
- Dollars spent per calories (1,825,000 calories/$6,133) = 297.5 calories for $1 (on average). We rounded to the equation that $1 purchases = 300 calories

We have discussed how to save ourselves and our families from the financial burden associated with the loss of beta cells by instituting financial incentives and motivations. Most of us may have some lingering questions about which factors affecting our family's health may simply be out of our control, such as our genetics. In the next section of the book, we are going to explore the role our genetics play in trying to achieve a healthy weight. Also, the neighborhood we live in may offer challenges to our family's ability to achieve good nutrition and activity levels. Concerns are now reported in the literature, suggesting that some neighborhoods have health challenges because of a lack of easily accessible and safe recreational areas, combined with too many fast food restaurants.

Do Genetics Play a Role in Beta Cell Loss and type 2 diabetes?

As in any chronic disease, including type 2 diabetes, there are both environmental and genetic components. Some body types are predisposed to gain weight more easily than others. In some native Indian tribes, scientists demonstrated that some Indians may carry genes that predispose them to a higher risk of diabetes. Also, ailments affecting our vital organs may induce weight gain or loss. This is why it is vitally important that we consult with a health professional before embarking on a new diet or exercise regime.

Which is more important, our genetics or our choices? Here is the American Diabetes Association statement on the matter (emphasis added):

> The <u>leading</u> cause of type 2 diabetes is <u>obesity</u> and lack of <u>exercise</u>. Since we often <u>inherit lifestyle</u> as well as genes from our parents, type 2 diabetes can cluster in families <u>even if no genetics are involved</u>. Genetic testing for type 2 diabetes is not available because there are so many genes involved. <u>A person could inherit one gene that places them at higher risk, but several others that place them at lower risk.</u> (Genetics of Diabetes)

Therefore, it is safe to say that for the vast majority of us at risk for type 2 diabetes: <u>we eat too much,</u> <u>exercise too little, and come from homes and neighborhoods where the same can be said</u>. Furthermore, we can also state that as we eat correctly and exercise appropriately, until we reach our healthy weight, we substantially lower, or eliminate, the risk for premature death of our beta cells.

Consult your physician if you are still concerned about a genetic link placing you at risk. After you receive their opinion, accept it and act on it. We all may need to practice better nutrition and exercise, regardless of our risk factors.

We do have some evidence regarding the nature of our physical environment, and how our home neighborhood may place our family at greater risk. We learned at the beginning of this chapter that simply living in America puts a person at greater risk for beta cell loss and the costs associated with type 2 diabetes. Are there states or counties safer than others? Please take advantage of the powerful government resources provided at the link below. There you can review the maps on the rate of diabetes by state.

http://www.cdc.gov/diabetes/statistics/diabetes_slides.htm

(Diabetes Data and Trends: County Level Estimates of Diagnosed Diabetes and Obesity)

The maps you will find provide information on the rate of diabetes by state and by county. Here is a sampling of the results of their analysis.

- The healthiest state is Colorado: Rate of diabetes is 15% to 19%
- Top nine unhealthiest states (in no particular order): Rate of diabetes is greater than 30%:
  Oklahoma, Louisiana, West Virginia, Arkansas, Tennessee, Mississippi, Alabama, Missouri, Kentucky

Based on diabetes rates, if we are living in the more unhealthy states, we have, on average, twice as many citizens living near us that have diabetes compared to those citizens living in Colorado. What is reported here is that we have entire states, with their communities and their families, at high risk for medical and financial catastrophe. How do we overcome a complete environmental onslaught on our families?

We must systematically build incentives into our culture so the epidemic does not entirely overwhelm us. The balance of this text devotes itself to cultural solutions that are available through our families, government, employers, healthcare providers, and insurers. These will all be addressed in upcoming chapters. Families in the U.S. cannot avoid this epidemic; it is systemic to our very culture.

Viewing the maps from the site mentioned above, we see that we are at higher risk from the financial distresses caused by diabetes depending on the county in which we reside. We double or triple the probability that we are obese or overweight depending on where we live and work. That means we also double the probability of experiencing the severe financial distress we discussed earlier in this chapter. Consider our individual family's incentives to stay healthy. How much stronger must we make these incentives in order to combat our disadvantaged home or work environment? Perhaps, compared to an average family, if we live in a high-risk county where the risk is doubled, we may need to double the economic incentives to keep our families healthy.

To begin looking at where we might use economic incentives, consider the study findings that discuss important elements that are close to home. These are namely, the ease of access to healthy exercise opportunities and the density of fast food restaurants in our neighborhoods. Another powerful map link is provided below. Google Maps gives us a fascinating look at the density of fast food outlets across the country by county. We can say that density of fast food outlets follows population density, as one would expect. http://maps.forum.nu/gm_heatmap.html

Scientists are now confirming that there is an overlap of populations with high obesity rates and with high fast food restaurant densities. Remember that *extreme* obesity puts us at a 700 percent greater risk for losing beta cell function and becoming a person with diabetes. These maps indicate that where we live may indeed put us at extreme risk for destroying our beta cells. Here is the proof:

A study involving 700,000 individuals found that: "Fast-food restaurant density and a higher ratio of fast-food to full-service restaurants" correlated to above average weight level and the risk of obesity [and therefore diabetes]. The authors conclude, "Hence, it is the availability of fast-food relative, to other away-from-home choices, that appears salient for unhealthy weight outcomes." (Mehta and Chang 127-33)

It is time to be direct. If we live in a high concentration fast food area, and we choose to eat at these establishments frequently, we will put ourselves and our families at risk for obesity and diabetes. To protect our families, we need to answer the question: what incentives do we have to not eat at fast food restaurants so often? Now we zeroed in on the critical question. If we think about it for long, we soon realize we really have little or no incentives, because the fast food outlets are close, convenient, tasty, and a cheap source of calories. To find the incentives necessary to drive past and not stop at these restaurants, we can follow the instructions and examples earlier in this chapter. They can help all of us battle the epidemic in our neighborhood. We must all put our own money where our mouths are, before the government must do it for us one way or another.

Before closing this chapter, all readers are urged to access the following reference containing further information on the risks facing some of our neighborhoods and communities. (Gearhart, Gurbur, and Vaneta 1-21)

Pointed out is the evidence of just one such risk, easy access to safe recreation. We face, in some of our neighborhoods, the prospect of our children having to stay inside our homes to avoid a dangerous environment. Factors that are found in these environments are high crime rates, challenging neighbors (drug dealers), and dangers like stray dogs. Both parents and children living in these neighborhoods find it difficult to find enjoyable and safe physical activities close to home. Communities can band together to vote for neighborhood improvements and greater law enforcement efforts to increase the safety and health of their children.

There is evidence that our lack of activity is a result of a sharp decline in the amount of walking we do on a daily basis. Americans have decreased walking by 42 percent in the past 20 years. (Chapter 2: The Dangers of Walking Less) Evidence points to the fact that those of us living in challenging neighborhoods are growing obese and killing off beta cells earlier and faster than our neighbors living in areas of easy and safe access to regular physical activity like walking. (Aguila J, Iturb, and Jackson 1-2)

In this chapter, we demonstrated the need for all of us, individuals and families, to step up (literally) and protect ourselves from the financial disaster awaiting us from our overeating and poor activity levels. We have also established the reasonable assumption that for most of us, we cannot get a handle on this situation without taking personal responsibility for our chronic risky behaviors. That responsibility includes creating adequate incentives to motivate us to reform our lives. Self-control and fad diets are not powerful enough. No amount of training, no amount of education, no diet plan to date, has worked to halt diabetes in our cultures. Why? <u>The economic impact of our decisions are not felt immediately, forcefully, and continually enough to prevent it from occurring.</u>

All of us can step up and use the incentives of EAC, or other ideas discussed in this chapter to build a happy health future for us, our children, and our communities. Communities are where our health can make or break us. In the next chapter, we will examine the impact our ethnic communities are having on our personal health, the decline of our beta cells, and the epidemic of diabetes.

Chapter 2
Reference List

Chapter 2: The Dangers of Walking Less. Surface Transportation Policy Project, 2011.

Diabetes Data and Trends: County Level Estimates of Diagnosed Diabetes and Obesity. Centers for Disease Control and Prevention and Division of Diabetes Translation. Centers for Disease Control, 2011.

"Disturbing Statistics about Long Term Care in the US." Mar. 1, 2011.
http://www.payingforseniorcare.com/longtermcare/statistics.html.

Facts for Families: Obesity in Children and Teens. American Academy of Child and Adolescent Psychiatry, 2011.

Genetics of Diabetes. American Diabetes Association, 2011.

IDF Diabetes Atlas 5th Edition. International Diabetes Federation. International Diabetes Federation, 2011.

Long-Term Care Insurance. ElderLawNet, Inc., 2011.

"National Occupational Employment and Wage Estimates." Feb. 22, 2011. Apr. 6, 2011. U.S. Bureau of Labor Statistics http://www.bls.gov/oes/current/oes_nat.htm.

New Factor in Teen Obesity: Parents. ScienceDaily, 2011.

Price and Taste Trump Nutrition When Americans Eat Out. ScienceDaily, 2011.

Aguila J, H Iturb, and E Jackson. "The Fattening of America: Analysis of the Link Between Obesity and Low Income". Stanford Medical Youth Science Program Summer 2010 2010.V 1-2.

Albright, A. Ann Albright Testimony. HHS.gov, 2011.

American Diabetes Association. "Economic Costs of Diabetes in the U.S. in 2007." Diabetes Care 31.3 (2008): 596-615.

---. Direct and Indirect Costs of Diabetes in the United States. American Diabetes Association. American Diabetes Association, 2011.

Bhattacharya, Jayanta Bundorf M. Kate Kate Pace Noemi and Sood Neeraj. "Does Health Insurance Make You Fat?" NBER Working Paper Series 2011: 1-42.

Booth DA, Booth P. "Targeting cultural changes supportive of the healthiest lifestyle patterns. A biosocial evidence-base for prevention of obesity." Appetite 56.1 (2011): 210-21.

Centers for Disease Control and Prevention. Diabetes FastStats.Centers for Disease Control and Prevention, 2011.

---. FastStats Nursing Home Care. Centers for Disease Control and Prevention Office of Information Services. Centers for Disease Control and Prevention/National Center for Health Statistics, 2011.

Christakis, Nicholas A. and James H. Fowler. "The Spread of Obesity in a Large Social Network over 32 Years." New England Journal of Medicine 357.4 (2007): 370-79.

Dall, Timothy M., et al. "The Economic Burden Of Diabetes." Health Affairs 29.2 (2010): 297-303.

Day, T. Guide To Long-term Care Planning About Nursing Homes. National Care Planning Council, 2011.

Dor, A, Ferguson, C, Langwith, C, and Tan, E. Research Report A Heavy Burden: The Individual Costs of Being Overweight and Obese in the United States. 1-27. 9-21-2010. George Washington University School of Public Health and Health Services. 2-22-2011.

Gearhart, RF, Gurbur, DM, and Vaneta, DF. Obesity in the Lower Socio-Economic Status Segments of American Society.Forum on Public Policy, 2011.

Godsey, C. Take-Out Foods, Restaurant Meals Tied to Obesity Trend. Kroger Health Guide, 2011.

Mehta, Neil K. and Chang, Virginia W. Weight Status and Restaurant Availability: A Multilevel Analysis. American journal of preventive medicine 34[2], 127-33. 2-1-2008.

Mokdad, AH, et al. "Prevelence of Obesity, Diabetes, and Obesity-related Health Risk Factors, 2001." JAMA 289.1 (2003): 76-79.

Shane, et al. How the Average U.S. Consumer Spends Their Paycheck.Visual Economics, 2011.

Spraggins, R. We the People, Women and Men in the United States Census 2000 Special Reports. US Census Bureau. 1-19. 2005. U.S. Department of Commerce. 2-22-2011.

Strong, K., S Parks, and E Anderson. "Weight gain prevention: identifying theory-based targets for health behavior change in young adults." Journal of the American Dietetic Association 108.10 (2011): 1708-15.

$$\Sigma$$

CHAPTER 3
Ethnic Communities

Soul food is killing our souls. Soul food is also killing our beta cells. Soul food is destroying the productivity of our African American families. The soul food that reminds us of good times, family gatherings, relaxed parties, and endless nights of laughter and love, feelings of fullness and satisfaction, is nonetheless destructive to our health.

The facts around this are unassailable.

- 50% of black women are now obese.
- 75% of black women are overweight or obese.

This is a national emergency of epic proportion. How is it possible in our technologically advanced country that we have allowed this to happen? How can we watch our loved ones slowly _**poison**_ themselves—and I use that word accurately? What is the poison of choice? In the case of soul food, we can all point to over exposure to FAT laden with cholesterol as a primary culprit. How can anything so traditional be so toxic to our families? For the soul of the matter, take a look at the table below. These are some common elements of soul food. Most, if not all the items, consist of 40% fat, if not more! Our bodies love the taste of rich (fat) flavor. Those rich calories touching our tongues compel us to exceed our calories for the day. Whamooo, we become obese—FAST!

Take a closer look at this cultural "demon". We term this a "demon" only because it is the ultimate irony that something we love, a joyful food, something that we associate with fantastic times with family and friends, may actually be a wolf in sheep's clothing.

Calories and fat content from Google searches, various sources including: (CalorieLab) List of soul foods: (List of soul food items)

Chapter 3

Table 1

Soul Food

Item – small serving Calories	Calories	Fat g	% Fat
Country fried steak	637	45	60%
Chitterlings	312	27	78%
Fried chicken	380	19	45%
Potato salad	462	27	52%
Fried catfish	314	14	40%
Fried muffins, Biscuit (two)	360	16	40%
Corn bread	290	13	40%
Bacon	90	10	100%
Pigs feet	230	14	54%
Sweet potato pie	340	16	42%

Definition of obesity: over 30% body fat for women and over 25 % body fat for men (Body Fat Percentage) quoting American Dietetic Association.

Soul food descriptions can be found at: http://en.wikipedia.org/wiki/Soul_food, which includes this ominous association with the death of beta cells:

> Traditionally-prepared soul foods tend to be very high in fat, sodium, cholesterol, and calories … In contemporary times, some traditional-style soul foods have been implicated in the abnormally high rates of high blood pressure, diabetes, clogged arteries, stroke, and heart attack suffered by African-Americans, especially those living in the southern and central U.S.A.

An important aspect of the preparation of soul food was the reuse of cooking lard. Imagine a typical soul food meal with country fried steak and gravy leading the pack. This meal may consist of at least 2,000 calories (probably much more, especially if dessert is provided). Soul food meals regularly exceed the entire daily calorie needs of an average American male adult. It also is almost 50% fat. The troubling aspect of eating these traditionally delicious meals is the terrible toll it is taking on our African American children. (Cristina, 2011)

> The diet of African Americans is particularly poor for children two to ten years old, for older adults, and for those from a low socioeconomic background. Of all racial groups, African Americans have the most difficulty in eating diets that are low in fat and high in fruits, vegetables, and whole grains. This represents an immense change in diet quality. Some explanations for

this include: (1) the greater market availability of packaged and processed foods; (2) the high cost of fresh fruit, vegetables, and lean cuts of meat; (3) the common practice of frying food; and (4) using fats in cooking. (Cristina, Garces, and Southerland)

As alluded to, our children at a very early age are conditioned to eat and enjoy prepared foods that are potentially harming them, if eaten with any regularity. We have established the fact that soul food is laden with fat, and when eaten in excess, can be toxic to the body. Before we die, the poison of overeating takes down our beta cells. Is this fatty overeating really harming us and potentially damaging our children? Again, the facts are unassailable:

For adults, this is what the carnage looks like right now: see Centers for Disease Control statistics. (National Diabetes Fact Sheet 2011 1-12)

- <u>African Americans women have a 64% greater relative chance of beta cells loss and diabetes</u> compared to their fellow American women.

We have previously outlined the tremendous economic downside associated with the loss of our beta cells because of our poor dietary choices. The downside is most dramatic in our ethnic communities and families. These families are all at substantially greater risk for:

- Reduced income due to chronic illness
- Reduced family wealth due to chronic illness
- Premature death
- Heart failure
- Stroke

- Kidney failure: As a specific example, please consider this sobering statistic. www.netwellness.org/healthtopics/kidney/faq2.cfm#b
- Although African Americans make up 13% of the U.S. population, they account for 30% of all kidney failure cases; 2-3 times the rate of the U.S. population.
- Cancer
- Blindness
- Amputation
- Reduced fertility

How can we stop this insanity of enjoying fat-laden meals? By putting our money where our mouths are. Before I explain further, please look at another rapidly-growing ethnic community, and their dietary choices.

<u>Hispanic</u>

- 45% of all Mexican-American women are obese! This is a 50% increase since the 1980's. (Ogden and Carroll)

How can this be so? Again, the Hispanic food culture bares the secrets of their sorrows. Mexican food begins with delicious and nutritious elements: rice, beans, corn, wheat, meat, lettuce, tomatoes, onions, peppers, and cheese. Due to the way it is traditionally cooked, prepared, seasoned, and served (in excess), this food has become extremely harmful to our beta cells, and our way of life. Although there is variation among Hispanic foods and cultures, we will primarily consider Mexican American ethnic food. Please review the facts below.

Chapter 1

Table 1

Mexican Food

Item – small serving Calories	Calories	Fat g	% Fat
Nachos	346	19	49%
Refried beans	160	3.5	20%
Spanish fried rice	177	5	25%
Ground beef burrito	430	16	33%
Chimichanga	350	21	54%
Soft Taco	170	10	53%
Quesadilla	520	28	48%
Chili Relleno	217	5	20%
Chicken Fajita	405	11	24%

Most meals at Mexican restaurants average over 1,000 calories—50% of our daily total—before you add drinks, chips, sour cream, and guacamole. Restaurant-sized meals for burritos, nachos, tacos, enchiladas, with drinks and chips, can easily exceed 2,000 calories—100% of the daily needs of an adult male.

- Mexican American women have a 66% greater chance of dying from beta cell loss and diabetes compared to Caucasian women.

Between 1988–1994 and 2007–2008, the prevalence of obesity among Mexican American women dramatically increased (CDC), from 35.3% to 45.1%. This translates to a 30% increase in the rate at which Mexican American women are putting their bodies at jeopardy for chronic diseases. If this is not a dire circumstance in and of itself, we must remember the children who are now faced with a dramatic risk of developing obesity growing up in our ethnic cultures.

Solving the problem

To find a way to attack this problem, we must feel the pain with every bite we take. This is the power of the economist. This is the muscle of a new approach: proven economic principles to help correct the environment in which we all live. To protect us from our culture, we need to understand that with every bite we take of our delicious ethnic food, there are biting monetary consequences, both short term and long term.

The following table summarizes Total Food Costs (TFC), for the average American family (2.5 persons), and adds in the medical costs of a beta cell challenged person(s) (BCCP).

- Total Food Costs (TFC) + Beta Cell Challenged Person's (BCCP) Medical Costs (see Chapter 2) and (Visual Economics, 2009)
- Total food costs (TFC) (eating out and at home) for an average American family (2 parents and one child):
    - ~ $6,000 per/year, ~$500 per/month, ~$5.50 per/meal
- Medical expenses for a beta cell challenge person (BCCP), where one family member is overweight/obese.
    - ~$6,000 per year   ~$500 per month ~$5.50 per meal

Therefore, Total Food Cost plus Medical Costs = $5.50 medical + $5.50 meals = $11.00 per family meal

The total food costs (TFC) tells us that for every meal we enjoy as a family, and one family member is heavy (a

BCCP), we need to include an additional $5.50 in our calculation of the true costs associated with average family meals. In other words, when we eat our favorite ethnic foods, meals really cost us twice what we think, if we include the medical expenses associated with being overweight. This is true for every meal, either eating home or eating out at our favorite restaurants. Consider the true impact of our eating by budgeting an additional 100% of the cost of each one of our home-prepared meals. The cost of each meal we eat at home is really costing us double if we factor in medical expenses associated with ethnic food. We need to set aside the same amount of money to pay for the cost of our diseases as we are spending to create our favorite ethnic meal.

Using this knowledge to prevent the loss of beta cells

How can we take this knowledge and put it to work for us? Our initial goal is to feel the economic consequence earlier and constantly in our lives to help us with our choices. The solution is to create a simple, but dramatic (>20%) luxury tax strategy for all the "junk stuff" items we eat that contain:

- No nutritional value
- 20% or more calories from added fat
- 20% or more calories from added sugar
- 20% or more of our daily recommended salt

All fresh, frozen, or canned fruits, vegetables, grains, nuts, meat, and low fat milk and cheese products are exempt. Any other essential, raw food group is exempt.

Implementing this tax system is easier than it seems. All food labels already state their contents and nutritional information, so products falling within the category above can be readily assigned a code for the luxury tax. Points of sale for food can conveniently report sales and collect taxes on the "junk food". All food taxes collected are to cover our medical expenses or subsidize fresh fruits and vegetables. Meal costs will remain the same for families as we move from junk foods to healthy foods. Demand for healthy foods will, over time, increase supply and drive down prices as production meets the new demand.

The impact of this tax will be immediate and sustainable. Parents will budget carefully and shift their purchasing power to supply their families with highly nutritious foods. Medical tax revenues will begin to cover medical costs. Medicare will come back from the brink of disaster, as we note in later chapters. Now, the obvious concerns: "why me, I eat healthily, and, can we afford this?"

To the first point: If no action is taken, we will all pay for the burden of our diseases by way of higher taxes/expenses. Explosive medical costs are forecasted. We either pay now or pay later. It is inescapable. Or, our system as we know it will bankrupt. Take your choice; do we want the pain now or the pain later? Later is not looking so hot. This action is a necessary result of our failure to place incentives into our culture to protect our beta cells. Incentives must be felt at every meal, with every bite, and with every purchase, or they simply will not work. Lasting behavior change can be reinforced throughout our culture and assist us in our attempts to eat a healthier diet. The history of obesity demonstrates that without financial incentives, education alone will be insufficient to stop the epidemic.

To the second point, can we afford it? Yes, because 80-90% of our purchases may shift into the non-taxed categories. As more healthy food and food stuffs are purchased, prices may initially increase until supply recovers, at which time, with ample supply, price competition will drive the price of healthy foods downward. Furthermore, as medial costs come under control, our taxes and health insurance premiums will decrease, providing us with added disposable income. In the end, this approach will be a net savings to our individual and country's productivity and health. We will finally put our money where our taste buds are. Some of us may even save our stomachs. Take a look at our folly: (Daven)

Quote:

> Today I found out that the 7-11 Double Big Gulp holds about twice the amount of fluid than the average adult human's stomach. The average adult human's stomach can hold comfortably about 32 ounces at any given time. (The Double Big Gulp holds about 64 ounces of soda or Slurpee).

These huge drinks are approximately $1.50! And may have 500 calories! This item has no redeeming nutritional value. With the suggested beta cell saving luxury tax, the government will collect $.30, enough to at least cause a burp!

We still need economic incentivized solutions to curb our over-consumption at restaurants. (Largest U.S. Retail Companies-Stores, Sales, Trade, Trends and News) "Sales at quick serve/fast food restaurants in 2009 were approximately $160 billion. At the end of 2009 there were approximately 945,000 restaurant and food service outlets in the U.S." We spend 30% of our food budget at restaurants.

It may truly take a dramatic tax >20% on unhealthy restaurant food to begin to cover the cost of obesity in the United States. If we have less money for junk, less junk will be bought. We will pay this tax eventually either directly or indirectly, due to increased medical costs, if we do not take action. Pushing it as a direct tax now will dramatically change behavior now.

The facts: The direct medical cost of obesity and indirect economic loss to obesity has been estimated to be as high as $51.64 billion and $99.2 billion in 1995, respectively; this rose to $61 billion and $117 billion in 2000. Researchers for the Centers for Disease Control and Prevention and RTI International estimate that in 2003, obesity-attributable medical expenditures reached $75 billion. (Obesity in the United States)

There is, on average, one restaurant and food services outlet for every 175 American families. With our proposed luxury tax on sugar and fat items, restaurant incentives need to be in place to fight the epidemic. Few of us have the willpower to resist the incredible edible ethnic food delights that are arrayed in front of us at our wonderful dining facilities. How can we not supersize when it is made so affordable? How can we manage our nutritional needs when just parts of the meal are 500 calories?

The simple answer, a consumption tax increase of 20% for restaurants where the average meal exceeds 1000 calories, and the food items that make up those calories have:

- No nutritional value
- >20% or more of calories from added fat
- >20% or more calories come from added sugar
- >20% or more of our daily recommended salt

How tough is that? Incentives must be felt at every food purchase venue to change our food culture. Walking into our favorite restaurant, especially those that are laden with rich ethnic foods of all varieties, means that we are spending a portion on taxes for not only our protection, but also for the health of the nation. We need to put our money where our mouths and stomachs are taking us. Next, try out this new incentive idea.

The Driver's License: Exam Question

Here is another incentive approach that is not as painful, but will yield dramatic results:

Incentive: The cost of your driver's license doubles if you do not answer this question correctly:

Question: If you drink one large non-diet soda a day more than your daily calorie needs, on average, what will your weight change be over one year?

Answer: 12 Pounds

Wrong Answer: I don't care

We want everyone to care. In fact, we want everyone to cheat on this question. Let everyone know the answer to this question well in advance of taking the test. A wrong answer may mean double the costs on our licenses, but eating poorly may mean doubling our medical bills at the doctor's office.

Here is an alternative question for those of us who are visual learners and butter lovers. (What Does 200 Calories

Look Like). Imagine, in your mind, two pictures. The first picture to imagine is a slice of butter big enough to lightly spread on 2 or 3 pieces of toast. The second picture is of 5 cups of bright orange, freshly sliced carrots. Question: True or false, does the food in these two pictures in your mind have approximately the same amount of calories? Answer: Yes. Both the butter and the carrots represent about 200 calories, or 10% of our total calorie needs for the day. Do they have the same nutritional value? The butter is all fat with no nutritional content. The carrots are low calorie and high in nutrition.

Asking these questions, with the economic consequences of doubling the cost of a driver's license if they are incorrectly answered, leads us to the area of effective education. Education by itself usually does not change behavior. To be concise, education, by itself, has failed to change our eating behavior as a culture. Behavior is improved by 1) changing our environment, 2) developing passionate emotions around the need to change, 3) increasing incentives, 4) having immediate and sustainable rewards, 5) preventing the loss of something important to us, and 6) education. Using these principles to our advantage, we may want to put some real spice into our driver's license exam.

The Driver's License Notification

The following incentive option is clearly more radical. It works like this. When you arrive to renew your license you are given a form that reads:

Upon initial enrollment as a Medicare beneficiary, if you are being treated for type 2 diabetes directly related to preventable obesity, the federal government is entitled to place a lien, up to $200,000, on your personal assets as compensation for your medical care. By signing this form you acknowledge this fact. Penalty for not signing: Driver license renewal is $1,000 per year.

Why are we so strongly encouraging this action? Why are radical incentives so important to consider during this phase of the epidemic? Please ponder the following realities for hundreds of thousands of our friends and neighbors.

The $40,000 Nightmare – America's Other Road-side Bombs

As horrible as war is, and it is horrible beyond description, we have a larger war at home with which to deal. This war is in every state in the union, and is growing out of control. There is no army powerful enough, no defense strong enough, and there is no treaty in sight. The carnage at home greatly exceeds what our armed forces are experiencing in the Middle East. The battle is with our bellies.

Please consider a very real situation for many patients with diabetes. They are unfortunately faced with the need to amputate their toes. Diabetes causes these amputations. In the vast majority of cases, amputation is completely preventable. Our ethnic communities are hardest hit by this complication.

- African Americans (eating ethnic food in excess) experience this surgery ~50% more often than their white neighbors.
- The average cost for diabetes related amputations is ~ $40,000.

- "Each year, over half of all amputations in the United States are caused by diabetes and subsequent complications, with most being lower-extremity amputations". (NLLIC Staff)

We are fighting a war for our health. Where are the war protests? Where is the body armor to protect us from this roadside bomb? Where is the dramatic leadership to organize the resistance? Where are the posters and placards describing this awful situation? Where is the M.P. standing guard over those who may inadvertently be providing the enemy's propaganda? What incentives do we have to win this war?

I can promise you that the patient with their toes amputated had no financial incentives in their life to help them eat properly and stay active. Just like the rest of us, there is nothing permeating our culture, from an economic perspective, to prompt us to realize that the cumulative effect of excessive chronic calorie intake destroys our beta cells and disrupts the blood flow to our toes. There are no compelling pocket book promptings, let alone barriers, at school, at home, at work, at church, at the movies, or anywhere in our culture. Common sense is not sufficient. Education has not worked. Who has the common sense to know that overeating will cost me my toes? Every year ~ 75,000 of us experience this outcome.

Although this story is too graphic for many of us, it does easily translate, and will cross, all social economic and cultural boundaries. For the 70-75% of African American and Mexican American women who are at risk right now, this war must be tied to the risk of immediate, substantial and ongoing financial consequences. We could lose our toes and our lives and our money and our property to an insidious disease, if we do not change now.

Remember the check from last chapter that we write, and hold to send to our worst enemy if we do not lose weight? A poster of an amputee patient may need to be printed and taped next to the envelope addressed to our worst enemy. The picture adds incentive to assist with changing our cultural eating menus and activity level. Next, write this statement across the picture: "Me in 20 years? Lose a pound a week". This poster may save us $40,000! The best return on any investment to date. If we do not lose the pound, send the check to your worst enemy.

May I suggest the following? We may all call this nutty, but we all may agree it would be motivational:

- Every home at risk (that is 2 out of three African-American or Latino homes), can create a poster of an amputee and places it in their kitchen at holiday time.
- High school and college health classes, especially those in a BCEZ zone need a poster graphically showing the results of an amputation.
- Extreme: every restaurant needs to post a similar picture along with their super-sized menu option. What if it is placed above the soda fountain for maximum affect? Remember, a supersized eating habit creates a supersized me, while killing all of my beta cells.

You think I may be kidding, but oh contraire, I am dead serious. The diabetes epidemic war is far from over. We must conquer this disabling enemy quickly. We need an all-out warfare plan with financial incentives for our ethnic communities in order to protect us from financial disaster!

Plan D (for Dialysis)

Plan D is for those whose stomachs cannot withstand the graphic nature of amputation. So instead, we will use something palatable. It is a machine. Study this machine. Know it well. It may already be in your life. It may be right around the corner, rolling in your direction. Find and print a picture of this machine and place it next to your bed, where the machine will sit for many obese patients who need it in the future. It is a picture of a home dialysis machine.

Diabetes is the leading cause of kidney failure. The increase in end stage renal disease patients in the U.S. was ~64%, while the population as a whole only increased ~10% over a recent 10 year period. If we lose our kidneys, we may need to regularly hook ourselves to this machine just to stay alive. The cost of this home dialysis machine is ~ $10,000, enough to buy ~20 laptop computers for our family and friends. Indeed, if we need this machine, due to our expanded and unabated appetites, our average annual medical expense climbs upward to an additional $30,000 to cover our kidney damage. (Morrison) The average senior household income is less than $40,000 per year.

Kidney disease is rampant among our ethnic communities, running 2-3 times the rate of the average citizen. (Demographics of the United States), (Rubin)

The number of end-stage renal patients has grown dramatically since 1996:

	TOTAL PATIENTS	ON DIALYSIS
1996	308,000	234,000
2001	412,000	297,000
2006	506,000	355,000

Source: MEDPAC; A Data Book: Healthcare spending and the Medicare program, June 2009.

I can just hear Patrick Henry yelling, "Give me freedom (to eat how much I want) or give me my machine." Patrick Henry was exceptionally talented in his truthful propaganda. Our modern day advertisers learned well from his verbosity. In this war, who is winning the propaganda campaign for our taste buds? "The average preschooler sees 642 cereal ads a year on TV. Most are for types with the worst nutrition ratings." (Hellmich)

The average school-aged child has never seen an amputation due to loss of beta cells, and most probably has no concept of the risk of overeating <u>in terms of the financial impact on his or life.</u> Although, they have seen many *robot transformers*, they have never seen a dialysis machine marching toward their parents' bedroom. You and I agree that no child has seen a fresh spinach advertisement sponsoring their favorite Saturday morning cartoon show.

Whose side is our friendly food marketer and manufacture on anyway? Do they influence our behavior? Do they have an impact on our purchasing trends? Why don't we follow the money trail to find out? (Story and French)

The electronic version of this article is the complete one and can be found online at:
http://www.ijbnpa.org/content/1/1/3

> The US food system is the second largest advertiser in the American economy (the first being the automotive industry) and is a leading buyer of television, newspaper, magazine, billboard, and radio advertisements.... The reasons that the food

advertising market is so large is that it includes the following: 1) food captures 12.5% of US consumer spending and so there is vigorous competition, 2) food is a repeat-purchase item and consumers' views can change quickly, and 3) food is one of the most highly branded items, which lends itself to major advertising. Over 80% of US grocery products are branded....studies of food preferences using experimental designs have consistently shown that children exposed to advertising will choose advertised food products at significantly higher rates than children who were not exposed;

Bingo: economics wins out every time. If we want to be part of winning in the food market, we must advertise, advertise, and advertise. Why? Because daily repetition with a positive incentive changes behavior, changes buying patterns, and is profitable. What a concept. We need to own our food marketing in our homes. We need to advertise to each other the good, healthy alternatives. We need to have financial incentives that we can rely on to help us change our behavior so that we too are making profitable decisions.

Ok, that's fine and dandy. All things work together for our good as we learn to flip them to our advantage. We now have another source of revenue to help us; in addition to the consumption tax, we now can suggest a tax on all poor-nutrition food advertisements that do not meet recognized national standards. Easy solution:

- ~50% sales tax added to the cost of purchasing the advertisement, borne by the food manufacturer.

- ~50% sales tax, borne by the food manufacture, added to the cost of purchasing the advertisement in markets with BCEZ zones established, and where the rates of beta cell death are clearly evident (see first and second chapters).

In order for the manufacturer to enjoy this opportunity to fully support their (young) customers through the cost of advertising, the food sold by manufactures must fall into one or more of these categories:

- No nutritional value
- >20% calories from added fat
- >20% calories from added sugar
- >20% of our daily recommended salt

This media bonanza sales tax affects all media sources, including:

- Radio
- TV
- Internet
- Phone
- Newspaper
- Magazine

To show a healthy respect for our beta cells, let freedom ring, but let it be bought with the price that is due. The price of killing off our beta cells is now off the charts. Let advertising budgets fly off the charts for products that, if eaten regularly, may do us harm. Let businesses feel the economic consequences of their decisions. After all, who can turn away a child asking for something sugary, sweet, and nice to eat? Not this grandfather. Not any father, or mother. Let us have a dialogue regarding who is protecting our children and who is not. Who needs to be paying for the consequences? Yes, we all need to buck up. We will start at home. But eventually, our Titans of industry need to be called on to pay their fair share when it comes to selling food that makes us fat.

Supplemental Nutrition Assistance Program -SNAP

Americans are so blessed. We are also so naïve. From the cradle to the grave, most of us are sheltered from the reality and consequences of our eating decisions. Is this unbelievable? Look at America's incredibly wonderful and hugely successful food stamp program, now called SNAP— Supplemental Nutrition Assistance Program.

Disclaimer: I love SNAP. It has eliminated hunger from a huge segment of our population. It means the survival for tens of thousands of families in dire need. It protects and lifts children at their most vulnerable moments. It is an integral part of our food culture and is a source of pride, charity, and good government. There is no "but" to this observation. Let's look at some statistics.

SNAP:
- Serves: ~33.7 million people, or ~8% of the population, or 1 in every 12 people
- Serves ~14 million non-children and non-seniors
- Serves ~ 14 million working age men and women
- A family of four may receive up to ~ $650 for food per month, depending on eligibility

Looking at this from an economist's angle, we find an average American family of 4 not on SNAP buys ~$800 dollars of food a month, including our food costs for eating outside the home. We also can calculate that every 12 families are now contributing enough taxes to cover one impoverished family's food needs (thank you). Each of these 12 families, on average, contributes $60 per month to help with food for the poor through SNAP. This is ~2.5 percent of an average US family's total income and ~8 percent of our average family's food budget. That is the power of the American dream and the American economy. All of us can prosper. All of us need to give.

- The amazing fact is that every family is now paying less in taxes to help the poor eat than we pay on average to cover the cost of our family being too heavy.

- We are paying less to prevent hunger and paying more to cover lost income and illness from our overeating. (Please see earlier information for statistics on average costs per family for overeating).

Perhaps the eating universe is in harmony – we are observing an equal and opposite reaction, the more we are able to give, the more we are able to eat.

Since we are talking about the laws of motion and mass, it is time we discuss bodies not in motion and gaining in mass.

De-acceleration: the Real American Pass-time

The following is *a Los Angeles Times* article describing a *JAMA* study finally establishing a healthy baseline activity level for most Americans. (Lee et al. 1173-79) The full article can be found at this link: http://jama.ama-assn.org/content/303/12/1173.short?home

> Most Americans gain about 1.5 pounds a year between age 25 and 55…
>
> The study was based on surveys of more than 34,000 U.S. women who were, on average, age 54 at

the start of it. They reported their physical activity and weight, as well as health factors such as smoking and menopausal status, over 13 years. On average, the women gained 5.7 pounds during the study.

Only those women who were normal weight at the start of the study and engaged in moderate-intensity activity an average of 60 minutes per day, seven days a week, maintained a normal body weight.... That amount of exercise is three times higher than the [earlier amount] recommended by the federal government -- 150 minutes per week -- to lower the risk of chronic ailments such as heart disease.

Now, think back to the 45 pounds most of us gain over 30 years since high school. This weight is 45 pounds of fat; extra, unneeded, unhealthy, simply unwanted body fat. All at the whopping annual rate of 1.5 pounds a year. Talk about a killer that sneaks up on us! This is the big one! And yet, it is infinitely small when you look at that pound and a half divided on a daily basis.

- For instance, if we eat all the calories we need for the day, except we eat an additional one slice of butter more than we need, we will gain one and half pounds a year!

Only 15 calories a day more than what we need—that's peanuts! Yep, two-three peanuts more a day! Tell me, where are we going to hide those two peanuts? We simply cannot accomplish our healthy weight and eating goals without incentivizing our daily activity level.

<u>Activity Level</u>

Using exercise as the base line, the average American adult, on any given day: (American Time Use Survey Summary)

- Spends 500% more time on TV than exercise
  - Spends 2 and a half hours (150 minutes) a day on TV
  - Exercises less than one half an hour (30 minutes). (Hours of Work in US History)

Over the past 100 years:

- Average leisure time per day increased from 1.8 to 5.8 hours
  - A net 4 hours gain per day
  - A 200% increase
- Time spent on meals remained constant over 100 years
- Manual labor, the majority of the work 100 years ago expended
  - 300 calories an hour
  - 1200 or greater calories more a day than our standard office worker

Our ethnic communities have expanded into the middle class over the past 100 years. Ethnic communities are now dis-incentivized to do manual labor because manual labor pays far less than an office job with a college education. This shift has occurred with a major change in the ethnic diet: more of everything is being consumed. More calories, and these calories are fat, salt and sugar laden. As a result, we now have the perfect storm. Super rich, fatty, high caloric food, all combined with new working lifestyles leading us down the path to today's early beta cell death among our ethnic cultures.

Economics in the form of capitalism provided this wealth of food. Economics provide the ability to work less physically, and eat more. Economics, again, is the driving issue behind our food excesses and will be the solution to our future health. We need to harness the economics of the modern day work life to help correct our cultural food excesses. What financial incentive do we need in our work life culture to help us move more? The next chapter will zero in on those incentives, and point us to a *lighter* future.

Chapter 3
Reference List

Hours of Work in US History. R Whaples. Economic History Association, 2010.

American Time Use Survey Summary. US Bureau of Labor Statistics, 2011.

Body Fat Percentage. Vegetarian Diet Information, 2011.

CalorieLab. CalorieLab, Inc., 2011.

Demographics of the United States. Wikipedia. 2011.

Home Dialysis. Home Dialysis Central, 2011.

Largest U.S. Retail Companies-Stores, Sales, Trade, Trends and News. The New York Times Company, 2011.

List of soul food items. Wikipedia. Wikipedia, 2011.

National Diabetes Fact Sheet 2011. Centers for Disease Control and Prevention, 2011.

Obesity in the United States. 2011.

What Does 200 Calories Look Like. Conjecture Corporation, 2011.

Cristina, M, F Garces, and L Southerland. Origins of the African-American Diet: The Afteraffects of Slavery. Facts.org, 2011.

Daven, M. The 7-11 Double Big Gulp Holds 200% More than The Average Adult Human's Stomach. Vacca Foeda Media, 2011.

Hellmich, N. Kids' Cereals Pour on the Sugar and Sodium. USA Today, Gennett Co. Inc., 2009.

Lee, I. Min, et al. "Physical Activity and Weight Gain Prevention." JAMA: The Journal of the American Medical Association 303.12 (2010): 1173-79.

Morrison, GF. Cost Associated With Home Dialysis. American Association of Kidney Patients, Inc., 2011.

NLLIC Staff. Diabetes and Lower Extremity Amputations. Amputee Coalition of America, 2008.

Ogden, C and M Carroll. <u>Prevalence of Overweight, Obesity and Extreme Obesity Among Adults.</u> CDC, 2011.

Reif, M. <u>Kidney Failure Among African Americans.</u> NetWellness.org, 2001.

Rubin, R. <u>How Home Dialysis Is Used to Stop Kidney Failure.</u> U.S.A. Today, A division of Gannett Co. Inc., 2011.

Story, M and S. French. <u>Food Advertising and Marketing Directed at Children and Adolescents in the US.</u> BioMed Central Ltd, 2011.

$$\Sigma$$

CHAPTER 4

Employers

The Lion and the Pea Shooter

The next important concept to consider is best symbolized by the king of the jungle, the ferociously fierce and hungry lion. Consider our situation this way: we learned from the last chapter about the dramatic decline of exercise. So we turn off the TV, get off our rear ends, and head to Africa on safari, the ultimate outdoor adventure. We are enjoying our safari on foot, when suddenly an enormous, hungry, man-eating lion, comes out of nowhere and charges us. Our only defense is to shoot it with the weapon our guide has outfitted us with—a pea shooter! If the lion carries out its intent, and does indeed attack us, what odds do we give ourselves for surviving the attack? Would zero percent pretty much sum it up?

The lion is laughing all the way to the feast when it sees the weak weapons we carry to protect us. The major issue we have with our safari situation begins with our naiveté and ignorance of the risks associated with stalking wild lions. The safari guide's motto is, "don't worry, be happy!" Eat and rest as much as you please. He tells us that the jungle is a beautiful place full of rich and salty smells and flavors. He is clearly living his motto and is not worried; given any danger, he can out run any of us because we have been sitting on our rear ends watching way too much TV. Besides, the guide can smell a lion a mile away. If we knew, with a <u>high probability</u>, that a hungry, ferocious lion was stalking us, would we ask some serious questions, like, "where is my body armor?"

In this story, the lion symbolizes the power of the problem facing us as it relates to our established activity/eating patterns within a food culture jungle. Everyone, including our exceptionally brilliant, talented employer, is informed of the problem bearing down on us. In the story, the guide represents our employer. All our employers offer us for a defense weapon amounts to a couple of pea shooters; simply no match for the enormously fast moving problem confronting each of us. As an example, please find below the current best suggestions, offered by the employer community, to assist employees with disease awareness and prevention. Ask yourself the question: where's the big gun?

<u>The Best Practices for assisting employees with their health</u>
- Provide a health assessments (health questionnaire)
- Offer healthier choices in the cafeteria and vending machines
- Provide nutritional information on cafeteria food
- Offer nutrition classes and exercise classes
- Offer weight-loss programs

- Offer health support via the web, and spread the word on good sites
- Encourage employees to walk and use the stairs
- Designate lactation rooms
- Sponsor health education lunch and learn sessions
- An allowance for enrolling in a health club
- Support community health events focused on weight management

(Managing Diabetes Complications: Focus on the Fundamentals of Care)

You are right. There is no big gun. As we shall learn in this chapter, we are handcuffing our employers from guiding us away from danger. In their quest to assist us, we put road blocks in the form of our lack of engagement in health initiatives, and our general annoyance for anything that is remotely close to breaching our sacred, confidential health status. To begin our safari, one that is hunting for real, meaningful solutions to the obesity epidemic, contemplate arming ourselves with some important facts.

- Most of us gain 45 pounds throughout our careers.
- Every pound of weight gain increases our risk of diabetes by ~2%. (Diabetes Prevention: A Unique opportunity)
- Over a 25 year career, the 45 lb. weight gain produces an ~**90%** increase in the risk of killing our beta cells and producing a retirement gift of diabetes or some other related cardiovascular disease.

In other words, most of us are increasing our chance of being eaten by a chronic disease by 90% over the course of our careers. All of this is now firmly predicted by medical science. What are we volunteering to do in partnership with our employers to prevent this poor outcome? Basically, we are asking our employer to provide nutritional information. This approach amounts to a sling shot—a downgrade from our trusted pea shooter. Who wants those odds? We need to beef up our protection, and this is how we can do it.

My fellow employees: ask for this action at our place of employment:

For starters, if we are fortunate to have a cafeteria at work, simply ask to eliminate all food on the premises containing the following ingredients:

- No nutritional value
- >20% added sugar
- >20% added fat
- >20 % of our daily recommended sodium

If we want something unhealthy, let's pay for it out of our hard-earned salary. If we cannot remove the food, double or triple the cost of all items that have the above content. Use the money gained from increased prices to subsidize fresh vegetables, fruit, and low fat protein sources or a wellness program.

Now that was the easy button. Here comes the information that will make us shake in our safari boots.

First, the facts, Ma'am

The average employee only pays ~10% of the total costs of their medical care; based on an out-of-pocket expense analysis (This is shifting up rapidly as this book is being written.). That's correct; due to our rich medical insurance benefit, we are shielded from the risk of our poor nutrition and activity choices. (Olsson et al. 1257-63) The very company that employs us and attempts to protect us from the damages of unexpected accidents actually underwrites, or promotes, a lack of financial accountability for our own heath. This is now called a perverse incentive. Not the kind we are looking for…. This is a true unintended consequence of our wealthy culture. Below is an example of how we can put a stop to this dilemma, at no added costs, except for that of our own increased accountability.

Annual Employee to Employer Letter

An employer truly motivated and concerned about protecting the workforce from the obesity epidemic may consider this approach. A simple letter is prepared and sent to each employee. The letter begins with instructions.

Instructions:

On condition of receiving health insurance at XYZ Company, just prior to open enrollment, each employee completes the following form. The information is sent confidentially to Human Resources where it is stripped of personal information and stored electronically in a manner that meets the highest federal standards for privacy.

Part A) Dear employee, please fill in the blanks.

1) I understand that XYZ Company annually pays ~$___X___ per employee to cover their employee and their dependents' health costs. (Amount X is provided by the company as an average cost per employee)

2) Based on estimates provided, I (the employee) calculate that the approximate annual medical costs (AAMC) for my health care, for year 20__ are: $_____.

3) For my dependents, the total AAMC is $_____, or $_____ for each of my dependents.

4) I agree with the consensus of national medical authorities, that obesity and type 2 diabetes are generally preventable. As such, the costs associated with these diseases are preventable as well. Yes____ No____

5) Based on national medical standards, I know my healthy weight and the amount of healthy exercise needed to maintain my weight, based on the food and drink I consume. Yes____ No____ (Healthy weight chart provided)

6) I know the healthy weight and healthy exercise needs of my dependents. Yes____ No____

7) To protect XYZ Company and its employees from hyper-accelerating medical expenses, I agree that excessive weight gain, non-medically related, is a legitimate cause for disciplinary action, up to and including termination of insurance benefits.

8) This is a matter of urgent priority to the company's long term viability and profitability. I understand that this issue is of utmost concern to each employee's short and long term health and productivity. Yes_____ No____

9) Signed by employee.

P.S: Thank you XYZ Company for your support of me, and my family, by providing us with this wonderful health insurance benefit.

Part B: Confidential

1) If not provided by the company each employee is responsible for paying for their own annual physical.

2) Weight, waste circumference, and BMI must be included.

3) Based on these biometrics high risk employees are automatically enrolled in disease management programs.

Currently, this approach is considered by many employees and employers as draconian and borderline unethical. To set the record straight, the "why" behind this action is supported by these substantial facts:

- The average employee with diabetes is voluntarily retired early at twice the rate of otherwise healthy employees.
- The added expense of producing goods and services for each individual with diabetes is ~$2000-7,000 a year.
    - There are over 17,000 firms employing 500 or more individuals, for a total of over 56,000,000 people. (Statistics About Business Size from the U.S. Census Bureau).
    - The author estimates for each one of these firms they may need to include a markup of as much as $350,000 into their total cost of production to cover the lost productivity and medical costs associated with diabetes in their workforce.
- The average diabetic is diagnosed in the prime of his or her career, >~45 years of age.

The above exercise demonstrates the need for employees to understand employer costs associated with poor lifestyle choices that most employees do not consider relevant to their productivity.

"Sugarization" and why employers are concerned for employees who are overeating

An unbalance between our eating and activity levels is creating a lack of productivity at work. Reviewed below are the scientifically confirmed clues pointing directly to the dangerous changes taking place in our bodies, without us even being aware of what is happening when we chronically ingest more than is necessary. (Brownlee 223-34)

Over time, as we continue to eat too much, we cannot store the extra calories fast enough, so our food circulates as excess sugar throughout our bodies. As this excess sugar circulates it gloms onto proteins and causes, in some cases, semi- permanent changes to our cells.

When this occurs, certain natural functions are endangered, such as the way cells grow and the way the body heals itself from wounds. In some cases, patients with diabetes develop severe wounds that may take months, or even a year, to heal. This is because the body's composition has been modified through a process which may be called "sugarization" (scientists use the term glycosylated). The average cost to heal a non-infected diabetic ulcer (foot wound) is $8,000 or $16,000 if it becomes infected. Increase the cost by 300% or more, if it ends up treated in the hospital. Yes, our employers should be concerned about our risky behaviors, including our excessive weight. (Kruse and Edelman 91-93), (Von Wartburg)

Also occurring in overeating patients is an increase in certain cells (cytokines) that can produce elevated levels of unwanted cells that cause inflammation. These cells have been discovered in surplus in most newly diagnosed type 2 diabetes patients, and are now considered markers for predicting the future presence of diabetes in those of us that have not yet been diagnosed. Preventing the formation of these molecules is a goal of some recent pharmaceutical research.

More telling, however, is the proven link between cancer and obesity/diabetes. According to the Centers of Disease Control there is an increased risk of coronary heart disease, stroke, high blood pressure, and cancers of the:

- breast (postmenopausal)
- endometrium (the lining of the uterus)
- colon
- kidney
- esophagus

(Obesity and Cancer: Questions and Answers)

No one needs to be told that these cancers are deadly. But we all need to be told that they may be preventable, and that the costs to treat the cancer are "sky rocketing". Let's just consider colon cancer, perhaps the least expensive to treat, and one cancer with a relatively high cure rate. (Chustecka)

> November 11, 2008 - The cost of treating colorectal cancer has skyrocketed over the past 5 years or so, and the costs of new agents and regimens have risen 340-fold, compared with traditional regimens. Although increased costs of treatment have also been seen for other cancers, the situation is particularly striking for colorectal cancer, say the authors of a report published in the November (2008) issue of the *American Journal of Managed Care*.

Privacy Privileges verses Employee Responsibility

No one wants their medical history revealed to their employer, especially if we are diagnosed with diabetes or cancer. We certainly do not want our eating and activity levels considered as part of our employment experience. Revealing our medical history is an outcome that is completely unacceptable. The purpose of this text is to convince us that the risks of excessive weight gain need to be elevated to the level of smoking and drug addiction, and that we need the same workplace incentives provided to address the plague of addictions, as we need to address the plague of obesity that leads to diabetes. Neither smoking nor drugs are tolerated on the job. There is good reason for this—both cause early death and both can impact the productivity of the employee. There is evidence that beta cell disease exceeds that of smoking and illegal drug use.

Consider these startling statistics for the United States population:

- Rate of illegal drug use in the United States is ~6%, declining slowly (Chapter 2: America's Drug Abuse Profile)
- Rate of diabetes in the United States: 8.5% (CDC) – *increasing dramatically*
- Rate of smoking in the United States – 20% (CDC) declining gradually
- Rate of obesity in the United States – 30% (CDC) increasing dramatically, especially in ethnic communities

The cost associated with treating and dealing with illegal drug use and smoking addiction is relatively steady or declining – while the costs associated with poor nutrition and activity are increasing dramatically.

Can we agree that it is fair, equitable, reasonable, and even highly appropriate for our employers to offer us healthcare incentives and benefits in line with preventing the risks associated with conditions such as type 2 diabetes? We are talking about incentives that are far less intrusive than a random urine test or a ban on smoking! Take a closer look at what we can voluntarily do to help our employers control healthcare costs.

- Volunteer to complete a confidential annual health assessment that calculates our risk of chronic disease and the projected costs associated with that risk. If the risk profile declines from year to year we can enjoy reduced insurance copay's and premiums. If the risk profile increases for preventable diseases, year over year, we can expect to pay for a greater share of our health care.

- Voluntarily assume the cost of additional insurance premiums if our weight is in excess of national medical standards. To work, this incentive probably needs to come close to 10% of our pay or $450 dollars a month. There must be a real bite out of our pay for this to even be worth our time to consider, or for our employer to engage.

- Volunteer to accept reduced copay's for office, hospital, and pharmacy benefits for those with a waist circumference (not waist size) of less than 38 inches for men and 35 inches for women. Exceeding these waist circumference measurements indicates a dramatic potential for disease. Accordingly, increase the copay structure for those of us not meeting these national health standards.

- Volunteer to be vested in retiree health benefits, only if we are within our healthy weight, the last 10 years of our employment.

- Volunteer to have union contracts re-negotiated to include increased union health benefits for those union members living within their healthy weight and reduced union health benefits for those members exceeding healthy weight targets, or for smokers.

- Volunteer to review a report on the cost of care associated with our family's health, by allowing it to be posted on a secure, password protected web page for us to look at each month. The personal health web page is accessed or reviewed prior to each pay day.

These incentives are non-obtrusive, both positively and negatively reinforcing, and can easily engage all of us that are employed in the problem at hand. How tough is it for me to have an annual physical that includes a form that it is faxed to my human resource department's confidential third party service, acknowledging the completion of the exam, and register my body mass index calculation. This is about as difficult as leaving a urine sample, or having my blood drawn because I fit the profile of a pre-diabetic person. Besides, if I am truly working on my health, this examination may possibly lead to decreases in my costs of insurance and to the cost of my healthcare. If we do not engage our employment environment with financial triggers, we are partially *blinding* ourselves from the harsh realities of our high risk behaviors.

What are the financial consequences of us entering retirement *blind* from a preventable cause like diabetes retinopathy?

Approximately 25 percent of all blindness is attributed to preventable causes, including diabetes. Elevated blood sugar levels eventually change the cell function within the blood vessels which supply critical oxygen and nutrients to the parts of the eyes responsible for vision. As the composition of these blood vessels deteriorate so does our vision.

Findings suggest an average of "$11,896 federal cost of a person-year of blindness for a working-aged American. Almost 97 percent of the aggregate annual federal costs of blindness... is accounted for by working-aged adults." (Milbank et al. 319-40)

Some reports indicate that retinal disease is occurring twice as frequently in African Americans compared to their white co-workers. In previous chapters, we have identified the underlying environmental cause for this most alarming situation. Employers can help stop retinal disease if we let them.

Screening for Chronic Disease Risk at Work

In the very near future, it will be possible to walk into our employer, roll up our sleeves and STOP—not go to work, but simply lay our arm on a device that can scan the content of our skin for signs of diseases that are caused by too much sugar circulating in our blood. Yes, that is correct. We need only roll up our sleeve, if we are wearing a long sleeve shirt, sit on a chair, lay our forearm down on a nice padded surface, and hold still for 30 seconds. Once done,

one minute later, the device will accurately spit out a one line report that gives us the probability of developing diabetes. It will give us a percentage, say 85%. This figure is based on thousands of users and proven biometric algorithms. The algorithms accurately state the odds that we personally have of experiencing the increase in costs, lower productivity, and shortened work life associated with a chronic disease. It helps us understand the risk of going blind.

This device may eventually be approved by the FDA and certified to be accurate within a narrow range of error. The reason the machine can calculate our risk is quite simple. Elevated sugar in the blood, over time, causes our body's cells to develop a different composition, including the cells in our eyes. That composition can be correlated to the amount found in patients with a particular disease. Once that is done and validated, tests are performed to verify the rate of these changes over time. Finally, based on our age and the amount of these changes seen in the body, an accurate prediction is readily produced. The cost to run this test can be split 50-50 with the employer, and may be as low as $5.00 or even free, if the employer is extra generous.

Car Insurance

Just like in the car insurance industry, perhaps we need to step to the plate as mature, self-sufficient, empowered employees and clearly understand our risk for chronic disease, just like car insurance companies understand our risk for accidents. Here is an empowering point system for us to consider. The point system below, modeled on that of the car insurance point system, is somewhat morbid, because it deals with our projected age of death. It may help us realize how our current health-related behaviors determine our long term future productivity with our employer.

Death Age Risk Profile Point System

Total possible points 5 – The more points the better

- 1 point - Completion of annual physical
- 1 point - Calculate ~ total cost of previous year's personal health care (my employer provides, web based)
- Plus or minus 1 point - Calculate my current projected personal age of probable death (5 minutes, this can be calculated from a number of free websites).
  a. Add 1 point if my projected death age exceeds the average national death age for my gender.
  b. Subtract 1 point - if my projected death age is less than the average national death age for my gender.
- Plus or minus 1 point - Calculate my ~ total of healthcare costs attributed to my over-eating (employer provided from readily available scientific literature; incudes certain chronic conditions, diseases, avoidable accidents, injuries and the cost of absenteeism. If it exceeds the company average:
  a. Add 1 point if the number is less than the national average for age.
  b. Subtract 1 point if the number is greater than the national average.

Scoring:

5 points = gold standard

If you subtract *any* points you are at risk for increased costs and lowered productivity.

This information is useful, and in many cases will be eye-popping. The score will not inherently change our behavior. But similar to the car insurance industry, here is the positive reward and the negative preverbal stick to attach to this scoring system. It is cost-neutral to the employer. The employee might want to choose from one of these two incentive options

- Those meeting the gold standard receive a 10-20% bonus to their monthly retirement contributions.
- Those who register a loss of points in either one of the last two categories need to, at their own expense:
  - Attend and lead workshops on healthy eating and activity.
  - Attend and lead workshops directed to preparing healthy ethnic foods.
  - Attend and lead educational workshops regarding health care costs, preventable disease, and the financial impact of an excessive BMI.

Employer Experience with Employee Health Engagement

The experience of some of our nation's most esteemed large employers points to pathetically low voluntary enrollment in health and wellness education (this is beginning to change). In fact, it was not uncommon to see voluntary enrollments below 20%. There are many reasons for this lagging engagement rate. Perhaps it was perceived by the employees that the information collected seemed something like a test, or similar evaluations, or an invasion of privacy, not a lifesaving gift of knowledge. The employee thought, "is my employer going to discriminate against me, or pass me over for promotions, or terminate me, if the information collected comes to their attention?" These are important employee concerns. We can address them firmly and positively.

Regarding potential for termination, the simple straightforward answer is no. It is illegal to terminate employment simply because of a medical condition. If the medical condition is known to the employer prior to offering us a job, or if we continue to perform our work within expectations after being diagnosed with a medical condition, our employer is required by law to make reasonable accommodations for the disability. Discriminating against hiring and against promoting qualified candidates with disabilities is clearly illegal. The laws of the United States support those of us with chronic diseases as long as we continue to do a good job, like any other employee must do.

Now here is the flip side. Does our employer have to hire someone who smokes, or is an alcoholic, or an illegal drug user, or appears severely depressed? No. Must our employer hire someone who presents themselves in the interview process as lethargic, low-energy, or in incapable of the physical activity level required by the job? Again, the answer is, no. So the bottom line is that once we are hired and doing a good job, we can expect that our employer is required to support us, and cannot fire us unjustly.

Will my employer inadvertently judge my work based on my weight? We will let the evidence speak for itself. We will start by reviewing a brief study about the general perceptions associated with weight, compared to disabilities.

In one study of nearly 3,000 people, obese respondents were 37 times more likely than normal-weight to report employment discrimination–not being hired for a job, not getting promoted, and wrongful termination. Obese employees are considered less conscientious, "less agreeable" and less emotionally stable than "normal weight" workers. (Kirkey)

Conversely, does it hold true for the opposite, do slender people make more money? Let us look at the other side, what is the corresponding advantage of being slender. (Bromstein)

Timothy A. Judge, of the University of Florida, reportedly looked at separate studies of 11,253 Germans and 12,686 Americans and found that women weighing 25 pounds less than the group average earned an average $15,572 a year more than women of normal weight. <u>Women's earnings diminished the more they weighed</u>. A woman who gained 25 pounds above the average weight earned an average $13,847 less than an average-weight female.

In this same study, men continued to make more money as they aged and put on pounds—up to the point at which they became obese—and then, compared to the peers on average, their earnings began to decline.

Perhaps we can reframe the way we approach this delicate balance of employer involvement with our personal health. Consider the possibility that there are no nefarious employer motives, only noble ones, the same motives that got us hired in the first place, and the same positive motives we have as employees that compel us to high productivity levels. These are the same motives that enabled us to be paid a good salary for the talents we bring to the table. The motives of our employer include the need to ensure the productivity of the associates; the encouragement for all of us to maintain our good health. Normally, the longer we work for a company, the greater our value and the more the employer's interests align with our own personal desires to stay disease-free.

Is it reasonable, or even appropriate, to suggest that when we voluntarily take on risks like gaining excessive weight or, even more wildly, decide to throw caution to the wind by participating in high-speed motorcycle racing without helmets, that our employer should support us without question? Perhaps we all need to ask our employer to help engage us in a way that secures us with both financial and health retirement strategies, and at the same time keeps our health status completely confidential. Many employers match our 401k contributions dollar for dollar, as the primary retirement benefit. In reality, our medical costs alone may exceed our retirement savings contributions from both our employer and our own savings. The following websites may give us a healthy dose of reality. To help us put our life risks into perspective, take a look at these websites and see if you can answer the questions:

- When will I die? http://www.deathforecast.com/
- Will I become diabetic?
www.diabetes.org/diabetes-basics/prevention/diabetes-risk-test/

Notice the percentage of questions that center on activity level, nutrition, family history, or weight. Our death is accurately predicted with very little information because these factors profoundly influence our longevity. A change in activity level, healthy weight, and good nutrition can expand our life expectancy by ~20 years or ~20%. 20 years of increased productivity, increased family time, and enjoying the fine things of this life.

Or better yet, if you are a betting person check out your odds at this web site:

http://www.funny2.com/odds.htm

Some highlights you might find informational include:

- Odds of dying from a car accident: 1 in 84.
- Odds of dying from heart disease: 1 in 5.

Or, looking at this statistic in a little different light:

- Percent chance of dying from a car accident: 1.2%.
- Percent chance of dying from heart disease: 20%.
- Percent chance of dying from heart disease is 17 times greater than of dying from a car accident.

At first glance, we may want to say to ourselves, "It is none of our employers' business how we drive, if we are prone to accidents, or if we drive in a risky fashion." That may be true to certain extent. However, many large corporations have thousands of vehicles on the roads, all driven by their associates. Do these corporations discuss the risks and hazards of driving with their employees? You bet they do. In some cases they:

- Offer driver training courses.
- Send regular news letters discussing such topics as the hazards of driving in bad weather, and the importance of regular tune-ups.

- Give safe driver awards.

What have these corporations found most useful in protecting their associates?

- Automatic employment termination if we are ticketed for driving under the influence.

- Instituting a point system for traffic violations, that rates us for risky driving and the odds of future infraction. If the maximum points are exceeded in a given time, driving privileges may be revoked and we may be terminated. This system is very similar to the insurance industries' rate-setting point process where our rates go up if we exceed the number of points allocated for a given time period. Rates almost certainly go up after an accident.

The analogy of driving a company car is important to consider from a number of vantage points. Firstly, we have employers directly involved in managing a common-day element of our lives (driving a company car) by using financial incentives. Driving a car in America is almost an inalienable right. An employer needs to be able to measure and, most importantly, put in place <u>financial incentives</u> to help us reduce accidents and tickets. Financial incentives change my driving behavior, not education.

Secondly, as my employer provides me this car, they are vitally interested in protecting their physical and personnel assets (you and me). You may be amazed to know that some companies experience an annual accident/incident rate of between 20 to 30 percent. Meaning one out of every 3-5 driving employees are involved directly or indirectly in a reportable accident in the course of the year. The repair costs, in the case of a self-insured employer, or insurance costs carried by the company, are necessarily expensive and are a major factor in overhead production costs. Furthermore, and more importantly, there is a huge factor of employee health risk, especially from an injury and death perspective. Thirdly, there is the potential for a major lack of productivity, as employees must take time away from work to handle vehicle repair issues and perhaps rent a replacement car. In some cases, third party vendors must be paid to assist the employee in the repair work and rental.

In total, employers spend a great deal of time, effort, and expense to protect us from the risk of driving a company vehicle. They routinely use financial incentives to assist in this effort, in a similar fashion to how car insurance companies manage their risk.

This begs the question, why would we think that our employer should not be involved in what we are doing to endanger our beta cells. On a daily basis, we are affecting the long term costs of production and our own lifetime earnings and productivity by killing off our beta cells. Just as employers are deploying safe driving incentives, and motivations to protect us while driving, perhaps it is high time to suggest that we ask our employers to become more aggressive in offering financial incentives that encourage us to remain healthy and to avoid chronic diseases. The Benefit Design Institute's, *The Towers Perrin Health Care Cost Survey* released September 28, 2005, showed:

- Employees are spending 64% more for health care than they did five years ago.
- Employer costs have risen 78% over the same five years.

- Costs for retirees under the age of 65 will rise at 10% a year. [50% every 5 years]
- 53% of companies offering retiree benefits are going to rethink their commitment to all retirement programs. (Rethinking Benefit Design: Innovative Strategies for Preserving and Enhancing Health)

It only takes a casual observer to conclude that most attempts at modifying our behavior and controlling the costs that are driving many employers out of the pension business are less than effective. To date, the literature is full of tried-and-failed, or at best, modestly successful programs that attempt to reverse the trend towards greater chronic diseases among the actively employed. These include value-based benefit designs and consumer-driven health plans which are discussed in some greater detail in the next chapter regarding insurance companies.

As employers rethink offering a retirement benefit, perhaps we can offer some financial solutions to further the support the case.

Take time to ask that:

- 401K contributions to be doubled for employees who are in their appropriate health zone.
- Greater access to be given to health spending accounts, so we can direct our purchasing power.

Let me end this chapter the same way it began: with the ferocious perennially hungry lion charging down on us. It is certain that we are under-armed to do battle with the beast that is our overeating and lack of activity. Most working Americans are simply failing at controlling their caloric input and are therefore failing to avoid cancer, stroke, heart disease, diabetes, blindness, and kidney disease, most of which is preventable and a direct result of our lifestyle. We need every avenue possible in our life to incent and motivate us into appropriate behavior. <u>We have the test of history that shows us that where financial incentives are absent, voluntary behavioral changes are slow or non-existent.</u>

We must hit ourselves where it really counts, in our pocketbooks, with tools amounting to more than mere pea shooters. Our employers are the source of our primary income and can therefore be counted on, with our support, to develop incentives that can dramatically influence behavior. Current voluntary education at work appears useless, because most of us simply do not opt in to participate. We stay on the sidelines. We can no longer afford halfhearted mild cajoling in the face of a national epidemic.

When the lion kills its prey, the first part of the body it devours is the gut. Why? Because it is rich with an overabundance of fat. This is savory fat, wasted energy saved especially for the lion's tongue and taste buds. Perhaps we need to rethink our priorities for staying well, to save us from the healthcare lions lurking in our future, poised to devour our meager retirement nest egg. We need to abandon our pea-shooter approaches which have proven ineffective, and embrace bold initiatives, the big guns, in the form of strong financially loaded incentives. These are motivators which truly have the power to protect our family's long term future and keep us from being devoured by the lion of obesity and the lioness of diabetes.

Chapter 4
Reference List

Diabetes Prevention: A Unique Opportunity. National Committee for Quality Assurance, 2011.

Obesity and Cancer: Questions and Answers. National Cancer Institute, 2004.

Chapter 2: America's Drug Abuse Profile. Office of the President of the United States, 2011.

Managing Diabetes Complications: Focus on the Fundamentals of Care. National Committee for Quality Assurance, 2011.

Rethinking Benefit Design: Innovative Strategies for Preserving and Enhancing Health. Health Business Communications. Managed Market Resources, 2011.

Statistics About Business Size from the U.S. Census Bureau. U.S. Census Bureau, 2011.

Bromstein, E. The Skinny on Salary: How Your Weight Affects your Paycheque. Workopolis, 2011.

Brownlee, M. D. "ADVANCED PROTEIN GLYCOSYLATION IN DIABETES AND AGING." Annual Review of Medicine 46.1 (1995): 223-34.

Chustecka, Z. Cost of Treating Colorectal Cancer Has Skyrocketed. WebMD, 2008.

Kirkey, S. Bias Against Obese People Increasing Study Says. Post Media Network, Inc. Canada.com, 2009.

Kruse, Ingrid and Steven Edelman. "Evaluation and Treatment of Diabetic Foot Ulcers." Clinical Diabetes 24.2 (2006): 91-93.

Milbank, Q, et al. Federal Budgetary Costs of Blindness. Georgetown Univesity, 2011.

Olsson, Jonny, et al. "Comparison of Excess Costs of Care and Production Losses Because of Morbidity in Diabetic Patients." Diabetes Care 17.11 (1994): 1257-63.

Von Wartburg, L. <u>Inflammatory Cytokines Carry Message of Future type 2 Diabetes.</u> L. Von Wartburg. Diabeteshealth, 2007.

Σ

CHAPTER 5

Insurance: The Forest or the Trees

A recent headline grabbed the nation's attention and sent shivers down my spine. One of the largest health insurance companies, in one of the largest states in the country, announced a rate increase of over 30%. This announcement serves as a fantastic primer for discussing the value that health insurance companies offer the market. Their very presence in the market place gives us tremendous peace and confidence knowing that we are protected against unforeseen adverse health events in our lives and in the lives of our dependents, if we are fortunate enough to afford their services. Health insurance companies and the products and services they provide are a vital element within our healthcare delivery system. These companies, at one level, offer a valuable service protecting the productivity of our work force, while at the same time attempting to manage medical costs. Due to mounting economic pressure, the notion of health insurance itself is changing dramatically and may not be sustainable in its current form as we all move forward into an era of extreme medical costs associated with our high-risk behaviors.

Historically, insurance was meant to protect us from accidents or random events. House insurance, flood insurance, life insurance, car insurance—all of these products and services are meant to deal with the probability of a random event happening. Does this same model apply to health insurance? The answer is yes and no, and this variance is at the root of tremendous costs shifts that threaten the private insurance industry all together.

Think of it this way: some health insurance benefits now pay for routine exams and checkups like mammograms, vaccines, teeth cleaning, annual physicals, etc. This is comparable to having an auto insurance policy that covers your oil changes, or a homeowner's insurance policy that covers your home air filters, or your lawn care costs. Experts say that these preemptive health costs are necessary to protect against even greater costs down the road or to help prevent diseases in the future.

There is sound logic in this thinking, up to a point. In reality, most preventive procedures do not control costs for a very important reason: they don't change our behavior. Think about the auto insurance analogy. Is buying new tires for our car a form of prevention of possible future accidents? Yes. Do we expect our car insurance company to outfit us with tires every time we may need them? No. Does the act of buying the tires change our habitual risky driving behaviors? No.

What is proven to change driving behavior? Answer: hefty rate increases due to our at-fault accidents and our speeding tickets. Preventative care or maintenance does not reduce risky behavior in driving or in our personal health care. Why then should we expect it to be covered as part our private insurance benefit package?

What is even more bizarre is our expectation that health insurance needs to cover not only accidents, but also our predictable health emergencies. Would we expect a property and casualty insurance company to write a new home owner policy for us right after we watch a television news program describing a hurricane that is heading straight for our home? Of course not. Then why do we allow ourselves the luxury of suggesting that our health insurance company must offer us protection when we are creating a high-risk health emergency by our consistently poor choices. Most of us are medical accidents already waiting to happen, and yet we say something like, "Yes, I may be 40-100 pounds overweight, but you, my trusty, loyal health insurance agent, need to offer me the same rate as I have always paid." These thoughts border on the naïve, and the thinking behind it is part of our health culture. This health culture can be summed up by, "Hey, this insurance goes with our jobs, and we are entitled to it for a reasonable cost, regardless of our personal behavior."

Perhaps this is why only 73% of the US population between 18 and 64 years old is covered by private health insurance. Unfortunately, that leaves 50 million people between 18 to 64 years old with no private health insurance and reliant on the mercy of local, state, and federal programs, or simply going at risk by not buying insurance. To put 50 million people into perspective, it is the equivalent of adding up the entire populations of the 25 least-populated states in the US. Or, consider it this way: 50

million is the population of Texas and California combined. This is the number of our citizens, ages 18 to 64 not accessing insurance. (Turner, Boudreaux, and Lynch)

Risking our financial wellbeing, and that of our family, by going without substantial private health insurance is not a wise course to follow. Recent studies show the dramatic effects on families that are unable to ward off the tremendous costs associated with health care. Medical bankruptcies are up by ~ 200 % (2001 to 2007). Some studies suggest that medical care costs and their associated burden play a primary role in personal bankruptcy court cases. Over 50% of these bankruptcy filings indicated that health-related costs are a major contributor towards the inability to cover expenses. Many of those declaring medical bankruptcy are working, middle class home owners, and most had some form of insurance, but could not cover the out-of-pocket expenses associated with substantial health care costs. (Himmelstein et al.)

All insurance companies attempt to control costs by reducing the amount of risk associated with the policies written. For life insurance companies, this means they measure our relative health and project the probability of our demise (how pleasant). With enough subscribers to their products, these companies are able to spread the risks across all policy holders and remain highly profitable. The same goes for homeowners insurance companies predicting the risk of burglary or fire, and for car insurance companies that have accident rate data forecasting costs. At the same time, life insurance companies will not insure you if you have a high risk health profile, nor will care insurance companies underwrite you if you are accident prone. Lastly, homeowner insurance companies will not cover you for fire if you are in a high risk neighborhood (been there done that).

Health insurance companies try to avoid writing new policies on those of us with preexisting conditions (that may or may not be the fault of our own behavior), and try not to renew customers that are perceived as too risky, and who are poorly compliant to their doctors' orders, as evidenced by their health track record. We cry foul to these industry practices, yet managing risk is the quintessential element of all insurance. Risk mitigation means reducing the risk from predictable adverse events. All successful insurance companies know that they must be excellent at this or go out of business. It is rational to allow our health insurance companies to do so, based on their expert financial analysis. Or, at least adjust their rates based on our health history and information.

This is critical to saving the concept of health insurance itself. We know that approximately 70-80% of medical costs are from preventable chronic diseases, and the majority of that is spent in the last 2-5 years of our lives. 20% of these costs can be attributed to diabetes and the death of our beta cells. It was previously presumed that most of these diseases were a forgone conclusion of the aging process. Not so, for we now know that many, if not most, of these diseases are from poor nutrition and activity levels, not from the aging processes itself. However, understanding this has not changed our eating and activity levels. From my point of view, only financial incentives are left as substantive options powerful enough to change our actions regarding our own health behavior. Insurance companies are heralded as a bastion of cost containment, and represent one such place where financial controls and incentives are a reality—so let's look at their track record for controlling cost. Does cost control come from the forest (insurance companies) or from the trees (the patients themselves)?

Managed Healthcare Dream

The concepts of managed healthcare and, broadly speaking, health care reform have tremendous, glaring flaws. The first, and by far the most obvious, flaw is substantiated by this theorem: Medical costs are driven primarily by poor patient behavior. Wait, this is shocking to most Americans. "How could the innocents be at the root of any problem? It is not our fault that medical costs are accelerating; it is the system's fault." Here is the list of the traditional culprits for cost increases:

- Greedy profiteering pharmaceutical companies
- Greedy and immoral insurance companies
- Greedy physicians and hospitals
- Under funded local, state and federal assistance programs

For 50 years now, insurance companies have had the great good fortune to have rich employers forking over ever increasing premiums. Where life insurance rates have declined as life expectancy increased, health insurance rates have skyrocketed. Managed care has succeeded, to a large extent, in developing models for quality measurement and payment schemas for reducing unnecessary and redundant procedures. It has also partially tamed the pharmaceutical budget, and ignited a standard for generic substitution for branded products. Managed healthcare, broadly speaking, has facilitated physician collaboration, integrated and standardized care, and begun to align resources in ways that favorably impact the care of severely ill patients. But, has managed healthcare tamed costs? No. Why? Because, "I am still free to eat, smoke, and drink whatever the heck I want,"… and at the same time have somebody else pick up the bill.

Despite managed care's mandate to control costs, U.S. healthcare expenditures have continued to outstrip the overall national income, rising about 2.4 percentage points faster than the annual GDP since 1970. (Managed Care) In total, managed health care has not delivered the model for cost containment for the country, even though in places like California, significant results are demonstrated with the pre-paid (capitated) medical groups and large managed care organizations. Kaiser is one of the organizations showing significant strides in cost containment, while leading the market in quality parameters.

The Kaiser Education Foundation produces excellent health education reports detailing quality and cost trends. A recent review of their well-prepared material produced a document that showcases, again, why managed care is not aligned to effectively curtail costs. Below is the list of "the major proposals to contain costs". As you read through these ask yourself the question, "which one of these proposals addresses the most fundamental aspect of cost containment—namely patient behavior." (Kimbuende et al.)

Major proposals to contain costs

Investment in information technology

Improving quality and efficiency

Adjusting provider compensation

Government regulation

Prevention: Proposals have been put forward to emphasize prevention by _providing financial incentives_ to workers to engage in wellness and prevention, in order to decrease the prevalence of these conditions and avoid incurring the long-term costs of treatment. _However, it is unclear how much prevention programs will decrease costs_ (more on this below)

Altering the tax for employer-sponsored insurance

Reported above are the current core proposals to help managed care organizations control costs. In fact, these proposals are reported by the Kaiser Education Foundation which has an outstanding track record of success in quality management. Of the cost control proposals, only one approaches financial incentives for patients. Examined closely, we see that these patient incentives are not deterrent incentives. These incentives encourage voluntary enrollment and participation in wellness programs. The extent to which these efforts will engage and change behavior to the point where medical costs are contained is inconclusive.

Since when is it the function of a health _insurance_ plan to actively recruit us to participate in, or pay us to attend, health educational programming? Can you recall the last time your homeowner insurer paid you to attend a seminar on how to avoid fire hazards or how to prevent a burglary? This concept is economically unsound. The point is, if we are acting in ways that increase our risk for damage, we will eventually have to pay more for our insurance – a lot more – or even risk not having access to home insurance at all.

These proposals, outlined by one of the most dominant managed care organizations in the world, demonstrate that, in our current culture, we are all grossly under-incented to maintain good health habits. After decades of trying to understand and experiment with cost containment and the drivers behind our escalating medical bills, few if any programs in the federal/state government or in private enterprise are addressing the real underlying issue—patient accountability. As a result, costs will continue to spiral out of control. It is time for all of us to stand and deliver the message that we, the patients, need to be counted into the equation of cost containment. We need to accept personal accountability for preventable health consequences and, just as important, we must welcome financial incentives to support and motivate us in our behavior.

We must contain costs or risk bankruptcy at a national level. However, politicians will not address the issue because they feel that to do so will jeopardize their reelection. They also have no precedence to stand on. Employers will not address the issue of patient accountability out of concern for privacy for their employees. We must contain healthcare costs to stay competitive. Insurers will not address this issue because they do not have a mandate from the employers to design the benefit structures that address the added risks we are all taking on. Citizens will not stand for it because it is meddling with our personal lives. Without our engagement, nothing will be accomplished and we can now forecast the demise of our standard of living. We have discussed previously how to empower our employers, ourselves, and our families to overcome this epidemic. It now becomes our duty to engage. The first step is to empower our insurers to support our efforts. Here is a plan on how we are going to do it.

Bright Ideas for Insurers: Cost Containment Strategies

Here is the big picture; just thought you might want to know, so you can now be considered better-educated on the subject of health care costs than the majority of your friends, business acquaintances, and family members. I dare you to call your human resource department and ask them what percentage of costs they think comes from physician and hospital services. 52% is the magic number. No magic bullet will control our behavior unless that behavior changes our need for both of these critical services.

Please review the list, below, of the percentage of medical costs for our system of care

- Hospital Care 31%
- Physician Clinical Services 21%
- Drugs 10%
- All others 38%

Example: The Heavenly Health Plan (HHP)

This example plan works. It is proven. Initial reports indicate that medical costs, specifically hospital and specialist physician services are reduced by more than 15% the first year and more than 25% off predicted costs the second year. The plan incorporates financial incentives for all stakeholders, including for the patients. The plan is sponsored by a large private self-insured company that saw the health premiums for their employees rise dramatically, so much so, that it impacted their profitability and was a contributing factor for a reduction in workers. The current cost trajectory for healthcare was unsustainable for this company. The Chairman and CEO asked a consultant and benefits advisors to develop a health benefits plan that would be out of the box and, at the same time, effective in controlling costs. This is the story of the creation of Heaven, where outcomes were favorable for everyone; hence the name the Heavenly Health Plan.

Initially, a health care benefit plan for workers and their families, including financial incentives, was developed. The benefit incentives for the employees were very dramatic, but right on the mark. Here is what it looked like in a nutshell. As an employee, you had two choices between a very rich expensive benefit and a more stringent inexpensive benefit. The rich benefit included total freedom of choice for doctors and reasonable copayments for office visits and pharmaceuticals but the employee paid on average about 30% more. The more stringent medical home benefit restricted which primary care providers (PCPs) the employee could see, and set high expectations for enrollees sticking with the advice and assistance of their medical home PCP. The cost to the enrollee was about 30% less on average than the other alternative.

Furthermore, and this is important, in order to access the stringent lower cost plan, the employee signed a contract stating that the employee and spouse would follow the medical home doctors' orders expressly, as demonstrated by making all follow up appointments and calling their health coach as recommended by their PCP.

The stringent plan included the stipulation that health coaching participation, prescription filling, and appointment compliance was tracked. These were reported back to the benefits administrator and patient in a confidential manner. If the patient failed to comply, that was ok; the first time their costs would increase or they would be transferred to the higher cost rich benefit plan, if breaking the contract rules continued. Let me repeat that, if the patient did not comply with the agreed upon care plan the doctor prescribed, the patient was automatically enrolled into the rich (more expensive benefit plan). Ouch.

Why was this ouchy? Answer: employee financial incentives, in the form of employee payroll deductions, are built into the benefit plan. Right from the beginning, during open enrollment, the difference in the rich and stringent benefit plans reflected real pricing in the market place for the benefits the employees and their dependents were to receive. Well, as you might imagine, during open enrollment most employees were lining up for the rich benefit, and then pricing was revealed. The rich benefit plan was 30% more expensive than the stringent benefit plan. Payroll deductions for the rich benefit plan design were twice that of the stringent plan. As a result, 95% of the employees elected the stringent plan.

At first glance, you might say, "This Heavenly Health Plan was over-the-top, and no one should be forced to limit their choice of providers—it is our "right" after all." Yes, it may indeed be a choice, so have an option to choose it, or not choose it. The point is, when you make that choice we need to pay for the difference. Chose the Cadillac plan and pay the Cadillac price. You see, the employer was paying the same for both plans. The employee was picking up the difference in benefit.

This is how the market needs to work to help change our health-related behavior. Employees chose benefits based on realized cost savings and quality improvements. What the employees did not recognize was that behind the scenes, prior to open enrollment, the insurance company negotiated discounted rates with providers that guaranteed certain things. The doctors guaranteed that they would follow closely the national guidelines for all major chronic diseases and allow their prescribing to be monitored to confirm they were following these predetermined guidelines. They also agreed to provide education for these diseases in conjunction with their health coach and to provide concierge level service including same day appointments, 1 hour turnaround time for office visits, and dedicated phone lines with answers in 3 rings. They agreed to follow national protocols based on proven science. In return, the doctors were guaranteed a predetermined increase in patient volume and payments per visit that would substantially increase their profit margin for primary care services. Importantly, if the doctors controlled medical costs based on historic data, while strictly following national guidelines for ordering tests, procedures, and medications, and achieving high patient satisfaction scores, they could earn substantial bonuses.

Now you might be wondering: how did all of this turn out? The Heavenly Health Plan delivered superior results and was a tremendous success. Here are some results: Medical costs dropped by about 20%, a big win for the company. Reducing medical costs was the primary incentive the company needed to develop this benefit design for their employees. Truly, this new strategy represented a big win, because during the same time period, community peer health care costs increased 10%, so the real difference was a 30% upside win for the company. The reduction in health expenditures allowed this particular company to retain the size of their workforce and prevented layoffs.

In the Heavenly Health Plan, doctors earned their bonuses, increased their practices, and saw better outcomes as patients became more compliant with their prescriptions and took to heart their medical advice. Most importantly, employees demonstrated an improvement in their chronic disease scores, as measured by lab values. At the same time, employees paid less for their insurance than they had the previous year. Yes, they were at first annoyed at the restriction in provider selection, but in the end, when the final survey of employee attitudes was assessed, the company was delighted to learn that employees felt they received excellent care. Quality did not suffer. Medical outcomes improved and costs were contained. All of this was due to financial incentives strongly encouraging better behavior of employers, insurers, providers, and employees.

There are certain elements of this case that need further illumination. The significance and impact of the financial incentives is critical. There was a tremendous dollar difference between the rich and the stringent benefit. There was also a huge difference in the primary care office service levels between the participating medical home physicians and the regular PPO network doctor patterns of care. It was a hugely motivating factor that rapidly engaged employees and created a new direction. This piece, the building of stringent health-plan incentives, may be difficult for many companies to swallow, and even harder to implement if their work force is spread thinly across a large geography. As it turned out, this health benefit plan design worked, in part, due to the proximity of all of the employees to the doctors that negotiated for the care of patients. Most importantly, it woke up the employees to understand the true value of their health benefits.

The full engagement of the benefit plan administrators in this endeavor was another critical factor. The administrators in this case needed to revise policies and procedures while allowing for radical experimentation. They needed to renegotiate rate structures, and in some cases, risk offending providers or other stakeholders that may have become disadvantaged based on the provider network that was established to implement the Heavenly Health Plan. In the end, the insurance company also made a financial decision—they could either retain one of their largest customers in this market, or lose the customer to a competitor that was willing to take on the challenge. The financial incentive was too great to pass up. They recognized the monetary opportunity of participating with this key employer. Financial incentives and a willing employer drove the insurance company to help create the new benefit design.

In this example, there was substantial risk taken on by all the doctors who agreed to accept this new health plan payment structure and deliver the enhanced service levels. They needed to redeploy office staff to handle their new patient load while at the same time closely monitor their actions to ensure compliance with national guidelines and service expectations. In addition, they needed to increase their patient-education efforts and record their recommendations in the electronic registry that tracked patient compliance to recommended follow-up therapy and education. The only way any of the providers would take on this added risk was the promise of earning a <u>large</u> future bonus if costs were contained (which they definitely were), and high satisfaction and quality metrics were achieved. They were happy campers.

The biggest winners were the employees. They were not laid off due to out–of-control medical costs. The company became more profitable and could retain their workforce. Also, they reduced their families' financial burden by accepting the offer to restrict options in favor of a lower health care cost contribution. Surprisingly, quality improved. This is a direct result of an ingenious financial incentive embedded into the benefit design, namely, "three strikes you're out". If you missed an office appointment, did not refill your vital medications on several occasions, or blew off attending a required health coach interview — guess what—as an employee, you forfeited your right to the inexpensive plan and were automatically enrolled in the rich benefit plan with twice the employee deductions, or you could opt out altogether. Not many employees encountered this choice (less than 1 percent); indeed, compliance and medical outcomes improved. All stakeholders won. This is why this story has a truly happy ending and can be called the Heavenly Health Plan.

Note: The location, circumstances, and results of this example are roughly based on real events. Due to ongoing negotiations, and potential conflicts of interest with all parties involved, the author is not at liberty to reveal more particulars.

<u>Heavenly Health Plan Principles for Success</u>
1. Develop a working team that:
    a. Determines the appropriate level of financial incentives.
    b. Ensures that all stakeholders have financial, quality, and satisfaction motivation.
2. Select an insurer that:
    a. Delivers on the proposed provider network contracts.
    b. Has a good grasp of these two drivers of medical costs.
3. Establishes meaningful incentives that are of sufficient magnitude to drive the behavior of all stakeholders
    a. 10% - 20% of annual income or profits.
    b. A fear-of-loss aversion component.
4. Develop a contractual employees relationship with:
    a. Options that binds them to follow the advice of the physician concerning the treatment of chronic conditions. The advice must be congruent with national guidelines and electronically (automatically) monitored.
    b. A company provided healthcare benefit with reduced employee costs compared to an open health plan benefit design.
5. Develop a contractual relationship with the employees that bind them to:

    a. Attend proven effective, doctor prescribed, in-house, or web based educational courses that are congruent with national guidelines, and are associated with their diagnosed chronic diseases.

    b. Automatic enrollment into a more expensive health benefit plan if they regularly miss scheduled education, lab appointments, prescription fills or office appointments.

6. Recognize that in order to control medical costs we must limit benefit options to those providers who will:

    a. Negotiate on price, based on the real potential financial gain for improved clinical, financial and satisfaction outcomes.

    b. Contractually commit to following national guidelines for prescriptions and procedures and electronically submit the compliance results of employees with chronic medical conditions.

Working with these 6 key principles and their supporting tenants begins a movement that will shift the landscape in favor of patient motivation. It transcends any current strategy in its effectiveness and reductions in medical costs <u>if fully implemented</u>. We need to ensure the rewards are real, concrete, immediate, and sustainable. We need to have immediate financial consequences for employees opting out, or opting to simply be non-compliant, with the doctor's orders. If a company can so shape their landscape, with the blessing of their employees and the help of an excellent insurance system, their increasingly nightmarish health premiums will suddenly become a part of ancient history. Next, we examine how these principles may play out in the life of an individual patient, for example, Gladys.

Gladys – predicting and preventing her risk for developing diabetes

Gladys is a college-educated, 41 year-old mother of 3, enjoying a middle management career at an accounting firm. She makes a good income and has, in the past, enjoyed rich health insurance benefits offered by her employer. Her family is extremely fortunate to have access to these health insurance benefits through her employer. Her husband is a self-employed contractor, and they could not afford the insurance offered through her husband's insurance broker.

Her main health complaint is that she has put on 30 pounds, which is about the national average for someone her age. Gaining a pound and a half a year over 20 years puts us squarely with this statistic. She no longer exercises and her family jokes about how all of them are becoming coach potatoes. At the doctor's office she completed a routine blood test. The doctor asked her to redo the test after fasting. When the results came in, the doctor delivered the challenging news. At the rate she was going, she would soon become a patient with diabetes.

Naturally, this came as a major surprise to her, and all sorts of alarms went off in her head. She listened carefully to the doctor. Gladys, he said, "Your type of diabetes is completely preventable. I need you to strictly follow my instruction because if you do not, your family will be financially impacted, and you could risk you insurance benefit altogether."

"What are you talking about?" thought Gladys. "Sure, I will follow your instructions carefully, but what is the deal about losing insurance benefits?" And then she remembered; during this past open enrollment her company drew her attention to a new copay structure that assisted employees with avoiding chronic debilitating diseases. She did not pay much attention since she was a clean-living gal, and in good shape, or so she thought. The new copay message went something like this:

Here is the list of chronic diseases that are generally considered preventable.

1. Obesity
2. Type 2 diabetes
3. Lung cancer (if a smoker)
4. COPD (if a smoker)
5. AIDS

Please take appropriate precautions to avoid these diseases. If you are diagnosed with one of them, upon medical review, you will be automatically enrolled into a new health benefit design plan. In this plan the following benefits apply.

1. Physician and hospital choice is strictly limited to special in-network providers only.
2. All scheduled appointments, lab values, and medications are reviewed by a third party to assure the employee is following the doctor's instructions.
3. Mandatory educational classes are completed at the discretion of the prescribing doctor.
4. All copayments and deductibles are increased by 50%. Maximum out of pocket expenses are now increased by 50%.

5. Failure to outright comply with doctors prescribing may include termination of insurance benefits.

Gladys reread, and reread a second time, this new health policy. She was at first offended, and in some ways felt discriminated against. She thought, "didn't they know that being overweight was normal in our family, and that we sometime even took pride in our rotund figures?" At the same time, she felt extremely motivated—she needed this insurance, and she certainly could not afford the increases in copays and deductibles. Good thing she had followed company guidelines and gotten her annual physical done. Without this early warning, it might have been too late to do anything about it.

As in the case of many patients, Gladys followed her doctor's orders expressly. The instructions were simple and included 6 basic proven effective actions, centered on exercise and nutrition, with the goal of losing 1 pound of weight a week over 20 weeks, or 5 months. Here are the actions she undertook:

1. At home, with family support, remove all non-nutritional food, especially those items with high fat, sugar, and salt content. Ask your extended family, friends, and coworkers to support you in your new dietary choices. Eat meals as a family.

2. Be active for 60 minutes a day, preferably with your husband or other family member.

3. Restrict eating out and, when eating out, only eat one half of the portion served.

4. Create meals with high vegetable, substantial protein, low fat, and low carbohydrate content. Expect to eat 25-

30% less than you previously ate at meals. Snack only on vegetables, fruits or nuts.

5. Drink plenty of water. Eat breakfast.

6. Get a healthy amount of sleep, between 6.5 and 7.5 hours a night.

Bingo! Gladys followed the doctor's instructions carefully and sure enough, the pounds slipped off, one pound at a time. At her next checkup, 3 months later, her blood sugars had begun to normalize and she had lost 12 pounds. She was thrilled, and her doctor congratulated her on this tremendous accomplishment. The doctor asked her how she had done it. She replied, "I made all of those changes to my environment with my family and friends' support, and every morning and night I saw the note on my bathroom mirror that said – you are so blessed to have great health insurance!"

This case illustrates the interactions of an outstanding insurance company, an enlightened employer, a dedicated physician, and an incentivized employee. In real practice, over 50 percent of employers are developing some approach to using financial incentives to help employees avoid the serious health consequences of contracting a chronic disease. Of that 50 percent, we really do not know the extent of the incentives--whether they are offering a $25 one-time discount to a health club membership, or $2,000 to maintain your body mass index (BMI) in a lower-risk category. We can assume very few, less than 5%, offer the type of aggressive benefit design differential described throughout this chapter. In the future, important work will be done to quantify what types of employee incentives really make a dent in the reduction of medical costs. For now, consider a list of a few of the incentives being offered by employers:

1. Points earned toward prizes for enrolling in a wellness program
2. Paying employees to walk 2 or more miles a day
3. Paying employees to get an annual physical
4. Paying employees to take a health risk assessment
5. Increasing the insurance premium for smokers
6. Paying employees to meet goals for blood pressure, weight, or cholesterol

What is known about many of these incentives is that they are powered to be too small. Their impact on employee behavior is temporary and transient, and they generally have not been shown to reduce total medical cost. The good news is that companies are beginning to get serious about this strategy in a manner that truly is supportive of the employees' attempt to get well and stay well.

Employers have stayed true to confidentiality and have not breached our cultural standard and legal policy of strict privacy in relation to personal health. This is the root concern for many employers and employees trying to implement these new changes. To help employers embrace this approach, new evidence is emerging that suggests that implementing a wellness program may be a strategic business move. Wellness programs support greater productivity and lower absenteeism. The most forward-acting of all employers on this subject are those that have been forced to address head on the issues of workforce health risks. Their senior management has engaged the issue. They realize their whole business model may be at risk due to dramatically rising healthcare costs. Senior management has determined that this approach provides a competitive productivity advantage.

As this evolving response to escalating healthcare costs plays out across our employer community, we can individually ask ourselves, "What is the upside of my participation in my employer-sponsored health benefit. What is the down side for my apathy on the subject?" This is a time to protect our jobs and our health future by fully embracing the new dynamics of health in the workplace. Keeping an open mind on new policies, engaging in the wellness programs, and expecting to pay more for our insurance benefit if we engage in risky behaviors, may translate into a reduction of healthcare costs and a more secure future for families. As we examine in our next chapter on Medicaid, our fastest growing public health insurance, creating new patient centric incentive strategies will be critically important.

Chapter 5
Reference List

Managed Care. Wikipedia, 2011.

OECD Health Data 2011 - Frequently Requested Data. Organization for Economic Cooperation and Development, 2011.

Himmelstein, D., et al. "Medical Bankruptcy in the United States, 2007: Results of a National Study." The American Journal of Medicine (2009).

Kimbuende, E., et al. U.S. Healthcare Costs. Henry J. Kaiser Family Foundation, 2010.

Turner, J., M Boudreaux, and V. Lynch. A Preliminary Evaluation of Health Insurance Coverage in the 2008 American Community Survey. U.S. Census Bureau, 2010.

Σ

CHAPTER 6

Medicaid Is Exploding

The rate of increase in Medicaid enrollment and subsequent diabetes-related state Medicaid costs are extraordinary. Former U.S. Secretary of Health and Human Services (2005-2009), Mike Leavitt, commented:

> The National Association of State Budget Officers (NASBO)… report should serve as an urgent reminder that the current path of Medicaid spending is unsustainable for both federal and state governments. We must act quickly to keep state Medicaid programs fiscally sound. If nothing is done to rein in these costs, access to healthcare for our most vulnerable citizens could be threatened. (Luhby)

Medicaid enrollment increased by ~20 million people between December 2007 and 2011, to almost 70 million lives. (Medicaid Medical Management: A Complex

Challenge for States 1-30) Over the past decade, enrollment in state Medicaid plans increased by 50%, while the general population increased by only 10%. Every year 1% of the U.S. population leaves commercial insurance, or the uninsured ranks, and enters the ranks of Medicaid. It now represents the health coverage for one out of 5 Americans, and one in 3 U.S. children. According to the *New England Journal of Medicine*, 16 million additional people may gain access to Medicaid via the recently passed Patient Protection and Affordable Care Act (PPACA). If this projection is correct, the 50 states and territories, in partnership with Washington, will now become responsible for financing and delivering health services for more than one in four Americans (not including Medicare, which will be discussed in the next chapter). (United States: Medicare Beneficiaries as a Percent of Total Population, 2010)

Chapter 6

Table 1

US Medicaid Population

By Age/Group

2007	US #	US%
Children	28,754,500	49.5%
Adults	14,627,000	25.2%
Elderly	5,934,900	10.2%
Disabled	8,789,500	15.1%
Total	58,106,000	100.0%

Source: US Census Bureau, Population Estimates Program
More Tables and Information: Population Estimates Program

Medicaid represented 14.8 percent of all health care spending in the United States in 2006. (News Release: Medicaid Spending Projected to Rise Much Faster Than the Economy) With some notable exceptions, expenses for healthcare for patients enrolled in state programs now consumes, on average, one out of every five dollars in most state budgets. Maine is forecasting that over 30% of its budget will be used to pay for health expenditures. In Alaska, the state Health and Social Service Commissioner reported that costs for Medicaid, "are increasing at about 14 percent yearly, and will reach $1.5 billion next year, up from $1.23 billion, the current year."

In Texas, the rate of Medicaid enrollment over the past decade was four times the rate of the population growth – (which by itself was twice as fast as the nation). In Texas, "Medicaid enrollment has increased by 78% in the past 10 years (growing from 1.9 million to 3.4 million recipients) while the state's population has grown 20 percent. Medicaid expenditures have risen at a rate between 7% and 9% per year...." (Texas State Government General Revenue Funding for Medicaid 1-5)

North Carolina, with a disproportionately high Medicaid population living with diabetes, reports that as of 2005, spending on diabetes alone consumes up to 50% of all corporate state tax revenue. In other words, North Carolinians may consider that approximately half of all the taxes paid by all of the corporations in the state are spent to cover the cost to treat patients in the state Medicaid system that, unfortunately, have developed diabetes. (Buescher, Whitmire, and Pullen-Smith 1-8) (Budget Highlights: 2007-09 Recommended Budget; The North Carolina State Budget Summary of Recommendations 2007-2009)

As of this writing, the state of New York is proposing 79 cost-cutting measures across hospital, pharmacy, long term care, physician services, and eligibility, to ensure that the state's Medicaid plan is financially sustainable. (Proposals Approved by the NYS Medicaid Redesign Tesm Feb 24, 2011 1-4)

To look at this highly explosive growth in Medicaid, it is important to drill down in the data to examine key cost drivers. Surprisingly, we find that diabetes ranks high in the cost category for Medicaid patients, in spite of the fact that much of Medicaid is targeted to children. Across the country, approximately <u>10 million Medicaid recipients</u> are diagnosed with diabetes. Using the previously determined current lifetime treatment costs for a patient with diabetes of $150,000, we calculate these 10 million Medicaid recipients will incur $1,500,000,000,000 or 1.5 trillion dollars in health care costs over their lifespan. As explored in our next chapter, this trillion and half dollar figure can be approximately doubled with the baby boomers now flocking into Medicare, as they turn 65 years old.

How did this increase in enrollment and medical cost occur so rapidly? Consider it happening this way: one patient, one family, one recession, one lost job at a time. Ted's story is compelling, and represents millions of Medicaid patients facing similar life experiences.

Ted's Story

Ted enjoyed a good life as an independent long-haul truck driver. That is, until he was diagnosed with diabetes. Then everything turned upside down. He did not crash his truck, luckily, but after feeling queasy, light headed, and thirsty all the time, and urinating frequently during the night, he checked into urgent care. Ted, unfortunately, was diagnosed with diabetes. To make a concerning diagnosis even more serious was the fact that Ted was an independent contractor in between jobs, so he did not carry health insurance. He thought he could make it through just fine.

Ted did not have the cash to pay for his medications, and ended up in the ER on two separate occasions due to his condition. What made matters worse was that he lost his license. Why? Federal law required Ted to see an endocrinologist (diabetes specialist), track his glucose for a month, and be relatively symptom free before he could drive again. The nearest endocrinologist practiced 2 hours away from his home, and there was a three-month waiting period before the next available appointment. By the time Ted finally was able to get the necessary treatment he had fallen below the poverty line, and became eligible to enroll in a Medicaid program.

It would be a year before Ted completed all of the rigorous requirements and paperwork (diabetes exemption forms) for his license. In the meantime, he lost business to his competitors. Then the recession hit, and a number of his customers went out of business. Ted, due to his illness, remained on the Medicaid rolls until his 50th birthday, when he began to turn around his health status by following his doctor's advice while simultaneously rebuilding his livelihood. Ted became one of the 25 million working poor, many with chronic conditions such as diabetes. Now he is back on his feet and controlling his diabetes. (Papp 1-12)(Diabetes exemption forms for intestate truckers)

Ted's story illustrates key elements of our Medicaid system. Medicaid is a life saver to millions of children, the working poor, the elderly, and the disabled. It is another mark of a civilized society, which at its very roots, protects American families, especially children.

Ted was protected and eventually helped on his way. What we see by examining his experience is heartrending. Due to his diagnosis of diabetes, Ted now has, what is termed a pre-existing chronic medical-condition. Depending on the healthcare reform, he may or may not be able to find affordable insurance for himself and his family. This diagnosis, in and of itself, may force him to remain under the care of the state.

Ted found it difficult to access the healthcare system to solve his medical condition. In many states, Medicaid patients are underserved. Only 30% of the Medicaid patients with diabetes report by laboratory analysis that their diabetes is under control. (Total State Expenditures Per Capita, SFY 2007) (Source: State Expenditure NASBO Report, Kaiser Family Foundation, 2008). Part of the reason for the lack of providers is that reimbursement is low. Too few general practice providers and too few specialists are available to deal with chronic diseases. In addition, there is a significant lack of education for ethnic members of Medicaid. Health education is sometimes lacking in its cultural relevancy, and may not be delivered, along with their care, in a patient's primary language.

Reports now document disparities across the U.S. among the poor receiving healthcare. One such glaring statistical example is that rates of preventable hospitalization increase as income decreases. The current CDC Health Disparities and Inequalities Report notes, "Blacks experience rates of preventable hospitalization at a rate more than double that of whites.... Also, uninsured persons are only about half as likely to have hypertension under control as those with insurance, regardless of [insurance] type." (Frieden 1-116) Conversely, Medicaid health benefits, considering the alternative of no insurance at all, are extremely rich. Providers of Medicaid services do a truly tremendous job with the resources they have on hand, and make every effort possible to deliver high quality care. They are true heroes in the U.S. healthcare system.

The issues facing Medicaid simply cannot be met with increasing taxes or generating more cash for the system. The perplexing issues confronting all of us must be solved through a combination of resource re-allocations and Medicaid insurance benefit re-designs that include appropriate financial motivation. Our healthcare system may need a remodel to keep up with the demands of this population, both in the sheer numbers of patients and in the tremendous diversity of patients entering the system. This remodeling can be accomplished through provider supply, patient accountability, vendor licensing, reimbursement incentives, and new care delivery modalities. These solutions are discussed throughout the balance of this chapter.

Market solutions to Medicaid's most vexing solutions: The Mary Story

Mary is a single, overweight 40 year-old woman with two grade school-aged children at home. She makes $7.50 an hour working as a retail clerk. She has trouble making ends meet. Her employer does not offer health insurance, and she cannot afford health insurance on her own. She is diagnosed with mild-moderate depression and diabetes. To find a reduced rental apartment, she moves outside of the city to a poorer, rural section. Her move makes it difficult for her to access mental health resources and medical care. Her mental and physical problems are affecting her performance at work, so she is constantly stressed about losing her job. She and her family are extremely grateful for the state assistance they receive for both food and healthcare. Due to Mary's chronic conditions, her medical expenses are above average.

Mary fits the description of thousands of Medicaid members. Perhaps we can examine ways to remodel Medicaid to help deal with Mary's health issues in a manner that reduces costs while improving her health.

Patient Behavior Generates 70-80% of Preventable Medicare Costs: what is Medicaid doing about it?

Fortunately for the general public, all 50 states in the union developed plans to address the epidemic of diabetes. These plans are readily found on the Web by searching the state health department for diabetes. The links to all 50 plans are also readily available via the Centers for Disease Control (CDC). States compiled their own unique action plans, all with incredible stakeholder collaboration. They also provide wonderful educational resources for providers and patients. Based on the understanding that the battle for control of this disease is going to take a multi-year effort, many states have multi-year plans extending out 5 years.

Here is a sample of some of the critical elements of these state reports. We can pull directly from the report table of contents, or, in some cases, the executive summaries, to get a general consensus of what the main issues are for all of the states and what they intend to do about them. The following is a specific example of a state report that is very typical of the many reports reviewed. Briefly analyzed, this report illuminates our discussion while making it more relevant. This information is directly from the state of Alabama. Here is the table of contents: (Williamson et al. 1-26)

Chapter 6

Table 2

Example of a Table of contents in a State Diabetes Report
Table of Contents
1. What is diabetes
2. Prevalence of Diabetes
3. Mortality Regulated to Diabetes
4. Risk Factors for Diabetes
5. Strategies to Prevent/Delay Diabetes
6. Complications and Costs of Diabetes
7. Preventative Care for Diabetes
8. Access to Care

Alabama, as exemplified by many other state reports, created a terrifically important report in 2009. They highlight the case for why diabetes is a health emergency for their citizenry. In doing so, Alabama, like most states, brings to life the horrific burden of this disease and provides free downloadable educational resources so patients and providers can take action on the information. Alabama went so far as to map the location of every endocrinologist and certified diabetes educator in the state. Remarkably, approximately 95% of the endocrinologists reside in only 2 counties and 80% of the certified diabetes educators live in only one county.

An important part of these reports, as illustrated above, is the Chapter 5, the section on preventing/delaying diabetes. Here is what the report actually highlights as the main approach to delaying or preventing the onset of type 2 diabetes:

1. Lose weight
2. Be more active
3. Watch your blood pressure and cholesterol
4. Eat better, more fiber, fruits, vegetables, and less salt
5. Stop smoking

That is all. It takes up a half page of a ~30-page report. The rest of the report, as you can see by the table of content above, is filled with important information about the disease itself. This is a fairly typical summary of all the reports reviewed. What is self-evident from our analysis is that the information in the state reports, and the actions plans associated with them, including: distributing education, increasing awareness, and provider involvement, community partnerships, etc., are missing a few critical and essential elements. None of the state reports reviewed for this chapter call out tactics that are <u>proven to help change patient behavior,</u> and neither do the reports offer proven solutions guaranteed to reduce the costs associated with diabetes.

Notice in the above, in the example of a highly typical state report, that the agenda does not have a section for either of these discussion points. One state report did go so far as to conduct and report on a patient survey that developed firsthand accounts of patients at risk for, or who struggle with diabetes. The researchers found something very interesting: <u>most patients already knew what they needed to do</u>. They just were not adequately motivated to do it. Repeating, they were not sufficiently motivated to change. The crux of the matter is not education, it is patient motivation.

States need to develop an understanding of what will motivate patients. In fact, when you really get down to it, perhaps that is all they need to be doing. Much of the education is already being done. The indirect benefit of figuring out the motivation piece is that once acted upon, cost reductions follow. We know empirically that when patients reduce their weight, through healthy eating and exercise, and stop smoking, that health costs dramatically decrease. We do not fully understand the behavioral incentives that provide long term motivation for the citizens in the state to avoid diabetes and its complications. From the reports we studied, it can be gathered that we have no formal action plan in most states to increase understanding of the critically important element of stopping the disease among our Medicaid population. There is generally no plan on how to motivate patients.

Discussed in the private sector is the encouraging phenomenon that employees can and do change their behavior in response to financial incentives that offer a 20%-50% difference in employee contributions to their own healthcare. Emerging reports may provide answers to assist in understanding how this approach may be used successfully in Medicaid. Some companies report that if they increase incentives, related to losing previously earned benefits, the non-compliant (high-risk-taking) employees improve their behaviors and their medical expenses decline.

These results are garnered by carefully incenting employee behavior through benefit design. Participating high-risk employees have benefit design choices provided to them that motivate them to control costs and engage in improving their personal health. These employees also work closely with their physicians to follow the recommendations found in nationally recognized guidelines.

This form of incenting behavior through insurance benefit design is missing in the Medicaid system. In fact, for the first time ever in the history of Medicaid, the state of Arizona announced a proposal that, if approved, would levy a $50 fee on Medicaid patients that do not follow the doctors prescribed advice to lose weight. (Adamy) This proposal was eventually eliminated.

The proposal was not just an arbitrary fine. It was a monetary incentive directed towards changing patient behavior that is risky and is found to be the root cause of many of the chronic diseases we have previously discussed. Many observers wonder whether $50 is enough to change behavior. It may possibly be, but behavior economics does not support the premise, because incentives need to be frequent, immediate and substantive to work. In the private sector, patients become more compliant if cost differentials for their employer-sponsored benefits are substantial. Healthcare benefit designs are successful because the employees experience the incentive at each point of care when receiving medical treatment (e.g. at the pharmacy, doctors office, hospital, lab, etc.).

Why are behavioral incentives not recognized as good medicine yet, and why are they just now being deployed in the private sector? These are curious questions in light of the fact that states bend over backwards to try to control costs through implementing and experimenting in managed care strategies. They have even introduced provider pay for performance incentive plans that have a modicum of success. These plans pay the physician a bonus if they meet certain pre-established quality of care goals. These physician pay for performance plans represent an entirely new segment of incentives in the market and are an experiment in cost containment. Here we have incentives created around changing physician behavior—but next to nothing introduced into the Medicaid market to motivate patients to change their behavior. This appears as backward thinking. Physicians do not create the original medical issue that drives costs—the patients themselves, in the case of preventable diseases, are the source of costs.

Earlier in this chapter, we discussed that New York introduced 79 proposals to control costs and reform Medicaid. Not one of the New York State proposals concerned incenting patient behavior around chronic overeating, and yet there were several proposals that introduced managed care elements to control physician and provider behaviors. From this action we may facetiously conclude that perhaps our physicians are eating too much and setting a poor example for the population.

When it comes to introducing incentives to reduce costs, we are generally still missing the economic reality boat because we really do not have direction on how to sail it. There is minimal scientific evidence documenting the effect of financial incentives on Medicaid patient behavior. The existing science is in the private sector, and points to the fact that some incentives do reduce medical costs and improve health. Instead of increasing the science around changing the underlying factors driving patient behavior, we are misdirecting the approach to the provider side, by asking the physicians and insurance companies to try to deal with costs. This is analogous to fining parents for their adult children's misbehavior. Our adult kids generally do not listen to us unless there is money on the table. Understanding the economics and consumer market forces that can change the trajectory of medical costs is in the best interest of all patients. This is especially true in under-resourced public health systems like Medicaid.

Now, to be clear, there are certain patients that are disabled, elderly, blind, or obviously too young for these incentives to be appropriate. Estimates put these patients at 10-20% of the Medicaid population. Perhaps we can work towards the 80% of Medicaid patients that have preventable chronic conditions, and design incentives to improve their behavior. We need to study incentives that motivate changes to patient behavior more than we need to study what changes physician behavior—we already know what changes physician behavior: evidence and money!

So let us roll up our sleeves and really help Mary, while at the same time decreasing her medical costs. We already provide her family with food and medical care, so it is a matter of helping her help herself with managing her diabetes and depression. A three-pronged approach is our best shot. This approach includes benefit design, touch points, and culturally appropriate education.

Medicaid Benefit Design Re-write, At No Cost to the State

In order to improve medical outcomes and reduce medical costs, Medicaid benefit designs may need to be modified for patients with chronic conditions. As a basic requirement to receive assistance from the state, these patients may need to enroll in a plan that includes the following:

1. Selection of a primary care provider
2. An online personal health assessment, reviewed by their health educator and provider
3. Demonstration of active participation in telephonic health education that includes compliance assessments of:
    a. Prescribed therapy
    b. Completion of health education classes pertaining to their chronic disease
        i. Conducted in their primary language
        ii. Available electronically
    c. Meeting mutually agreed upon weight loss goals (one to two pounds a month)
4. Compliance to their individual treatment plan allows the state to continue to have a no-copay benefit design

    a. Non-compliance status, first year: 10% copay collected, at point of care

    b. Non-compliance status, second year: $500 initial deductible, and 20% copay collected at point of care

State and federal governments routinely collect fees for non-compliance to state law. Increasing the cost of Medicaid benefits for individual patient non-compliance is rational, supports patient health, aligns incentives, and results in less medical costs. Programs similar to this one, completed in the private market, show a positive return on investment (Pomerantz, Toney, and Hill 137-42)

In Mary's case, special consideration for the diagnosis and treatment of depression may need some additional underscoring. Behavior challenges, like depression, prevent patients from setting and accomplishing personal goals, and need to be addressed early on in the treatment plan. Frequent, brief, telephonic communication from health educators positively reinforces treatment goals and objectives. They also assist patients with the day-to-day challenges of compliance and persistency with their doctor's treatment plan for them.

All desired permanent behavioral change needs frequent, long-term reinforcement. New technologies allow us to engage the patient regularly to ensure their healthy trends are sustained. Also, personal health risk assessments (HRA) are a beneficial tool (Plexcia, Herrick, and Chavis 1678-84) for earlier identification of health problems, making cost-effective interventions possible. HRA's alone may help reduce long-term health expenses. To reiterate, telephonic educational interventions coordinated with the primary care provider, with compliance to specific treatment plans, result in positive outcomes. Patients may be identified as a result of HRA's uncovering a high-risk health condition. The programs for these patients, if engaged early with the proper incentive benefit design, may show a positive return on investment and a reduction in overall medical costs. These programs increase healthy behaviors in patients while decreasing future healthcare liabilities. State Medicaid plans need both of these results to occur regularly in their patient populations.

Long term issues for Mary may include job training that can raise her and her family out of poverty. An analysis of job training policy goes beyond the scope of our discussion. Suffice it to say that a state university education needs to quickly evolve into online solutions, so that costs can be dramatically reduced. Medicaid may directly benefit by increasing the graduation of more health care workers—perhaps assisted originally by a revised Medicaid incentive system that can reward patients for pursuing their occupational education.

As it turns out, Mary did very well in this new Medicaid benefit design world. Through taking the HRA, Mary gained a greater understanding of the health risks she and her family were facing with her mild to moderate depression and her uncontrolled diabetes. She responded to the loss-aversion nature of the new copay design that required her to be compliant with provider directions in order to avoid copays.

Mary gained nutrition and exercise strategies and life skills by participating in the mandatory online learning prescribed by her diagnosing physician. The education was culturally appropriate, so she could relate to and implement the needed changes to her environment. She gradually lost weight over time, got her diabetes under control and completed her online Associate degree in health education. All of this was conveniently arranged for her with assistance from the state. Mary was able to double her income, and gain employment with a company that provided health insurance. In her new career, she began to educate others using her life experience as well as her new degreed education. She is grateful that the state was there to assist her and her family.

Much of Mary's treatment plan was successfully followed, due to advancements in motivational benefit designs that incorporate internet and cellular technologies. She frequently received brief phone calls or texts from her health educator, was able to take online courses to earn a degree, and complete state-mandated education prescribed by her provider for both depression and diabetes. This coursework was part of the requirement for her to remain in the low-cost copay structure offered by the state Medicaid plan.

The life skills she developed through this coursework, along with the Associate degree technical training, helped put her on a path to independence. When asked what made the difference in her success, Mary reported that the financial incentives requiring behavioral change were very motivating. Mary's situation and her life's direction improved due to a new state benefit design that incentivized her healthy behavior.

The science supporting financial incentives as applied to healthcare is just now making its way into the literature.

Research pertaining to improving patient behavior, specifically relating to the patient's ability to, over the long run, lower their health risk factors, is minimal. Consider looking at it this way. Imagine your grandmother, 40 years ago, going to the doctor and hearing the words from her doctor: "Now, if you are good about following my directions, you can earn some extra points towards purchasing something in the pharmacy that you may need later on." This seems almost whimsical, and yet this very action is part of an initial pilot project in Florida, testing the theory that awarding a patient for health-related behavior may increase their healthy actions.

The great advancement taking place, due in part to the new healthcare legislation, is that the Federal government recognizes the fact that financial incentives may soon need to play a substantial role in helping change patient behavior. This is being demonstrated on a larger scale most recently with many self-insured U.S. corporations. Unfortunately, the methodology in the state government experiment is severely restricted by the size and frequency of the behavioral reward. In other words, the Florida patient cannot earn a Cadillac as a prize. The patient is limited to receiving around $125 dollars in value. That is less than $0.30 cents a day in value. Imagine changing our behavior based on a financial incentive that represents approximately one third of one percent (.003) of our income or the equivalent of 3 sticks of gum. After all, what does it take to lose that extra 40 pounds floating around our midriffs? The private sector corporations studying the differential effect of patient health incentives are doing so at a much greater magnitude—nearly five to ten times the incentive amount currently under consideration for Medicaid patients.

Other states besides Florida are experimenting in this area, including Idaho, and West Virginia. Some states even have punitive disincentives. These states restrict access to additional education or products if certain behavior changes are not demonstrated by patients. Some of these approaches seem to be counterproductive and appear to generate negative responses. In addition, to date, enrollment in these state programs is lackluster, and there remains limited evidence that they decrease costs and increase quality. The majority of the increased benefit (reward) to the participating Florida Medicaid patients is earned if the patient simply makes it to a scheduled provider appointment.

There are the differences between Mary's experience in our example above, and these state health motivation tactics. The differences are subtle, but very important. Mary's new Medicaid benefit design does not reward her with additional redeemable credits or cash equivalent perks. In our example, Mary's state Medicaid benefit design increases copays to help her understand that she may loss benefits, if she does not make behavioral changes.

We can look at the example benefit re-design in two ways. We may view it as punitive in nature, because Mary will need to come up with dollars to cover the increase in copays if she remains unmotivated. Or, we can define this strategy, in behavioral economics terms, as a loss-preventive incentive. Mary is motivated, not in a hope-to-gain situation, but with a fear-of-loss scenario. "I do not want to lose my copay waiver," she said.

This distinction is critically essential. We know, from a behavioral science standpoint, that a fear-of-loss motivation causes a two to six-fold increase in desired outcomes. The health benefits, which she uses regularly and are of critical importance to her, may be lost (or downgraded) if she fails to follow her prescribed treatment plan. Mary responded positively to this motivation and was fully engaged. Possible loss of her benefits meant 1,000's of dollars to her. This was 10 to 20 times more motivating than the hope of gaining a freebie from the pharmacy, as in the real-life Medicaid pilot study.

Researching magnitude and frequency of financial incentives for Medicaid patients will eventually lead to a positive upside on patient health through improved patient adherence to their treatment plan. Figuring out this framework is well worth our time and tax dollars. Take a look at how patients that are compliant to their treatment plan improve their health in a clinical trial that includes a control group. This is found in the *New England Journal of Medicine*. (Chamberlain and DeMorey)

Diet and exercise that achieved a 5- to 7-percent weight loss [in study participants] reduced diabetes incidence by 58 percent in participants randomized to the study's lifestyle intervention group. Participants in this group exercised at moderate intensity, usually by walking an average of 30 minutes a day five days a week, and lowered their intake of fat and calories.... Participants in the lifestyle intervention arm received training in diet, exercise (most chose walking), and behavior modification skills.

A 58% reduction in patients developing diabetes seems evidence enough for us to gain this advantage. The key points are:

1. Enroll in a clinical trial [benefit design], where your performance is:
   a. Measured
   b. Reported
2. Walk 30 minutes a day
3. Lower fat and overall calorie intake
4. Attend training in diet, exercise, and behavior modification skills

In our example, Mary our Medicaid patient basically enrolled in a trial when she accepted the Medicaid benefit design of 1) no copays and 2) documenting and tracking her behavior changes. Reporting her progress regularly to a health educator and receiving proven training techniques on behavior modification, nutrition, and exercise put Mary in a position where she could enjoy a winning outcome.

Incentives sufficient to change our behaviors are not a matter of rocket science, but more of ferreting out the science that demonstrates results. Initiatives that have been proven to be insufficient, or are flat out unsuccessful, need to be abandoned like a used booster rocket. Most patient incentives in Medicaid are too small to succeed. Incentives that are too small may be inadvertently created out of legitimate concerns for patient safety, care quality, or just to avoid potentially unethical situations, including unintended consequences. These concerns are real and appropriate.

What remains is the evidence that current Medicaid health benefit incentives are generally not impactful or meaningful to patients, as they themselves report. Nor are they supported with regular training and the appropriate level of reinforcements. As an example, very few of the Florida Medicaid patients volunteered to go to the weight management classes—why?—because there was nothing in it for them for the long term. The incentive to attend the class was simply too small, and inconsequential. At best, these patients may have been able to earn 50 points to use towards a pharmacy purchase.

Models in the private sector suggest that these incentives would need to be 10 times that size, and shaped into a loss-aversion incentive, as opposed to a hope-to-gain strategy. Loss aversion is exemplified when we are concerned that something we already possess may be lost, if we do not take some well-defined action. We demonstrated in our example of Mary above, that concern over losing the copay benefit she already was entitled to receive was a positive motivational force in her life. This example includes a motivational force strong enough to encourage a Medicaid patient to follow a well-defined, physician directed treatment plan.

Fortunately for all us, there is a new round of federally funded Medicaid projects—in the order of $100,000,000, as part of the new healthcare legislation. This funding, in the form of federal grants, is specifically designed for states to implement new motivational strategies with their patients. The information derived from the results of these block grants will again point us further down the road to a place where we can understand what type of incentives, including loss aversion, may genuinely encourage sustainable and effective behavior change in this important Medicaid population.

Before we conclude this chapter, it may be important to consider how we can implement these new motivations, without increasing costs. Or how, in fact, we may even be able to decrease health care costs by their effective use. Telehealth and telemedicine are rapidly evolving areas of benefit design, and may offer promising results in this important endeavor. Telehealth is a broad category of how to effectively communicate health information to patients via the internet or phone, etc. Telemedicine seems to encompass similar tactics but may also include remote prescribing and remote appointments with providers. Without implementing new reimbursement strategies supporting more widespread use and standardization protocols around the use of this technology, the adoption curve for this approach to medical care may dramatically slow down.

Many states are progressive in this area. Check with your individual state Medicaid program for details. To date:

> It's up to each state to specify what telemedicine/telehealth services, if any, are eligible for Medicaid reimbursement. For states that do offer telehealth reimbursement under Medicaid, relevant issues impacting reimbursement include: Does therapy fall under the state's Medicaid covered services (or is it an optional service)? Are psychologists included in the state's Medicaid list of qualifying providers? ...Medicaid reimbursement for telehealth services by psychologists is available in as many as 13 states.... Coverage and billing requirements vary by state. (Legal & Regulatory Affairs Staff)

To secure our future with Medicaid, we need to control costs and bend the diabetes epidemic curve so that it is heading south. We are mastering a tremendous amount of information at a state level regarding the impact, the demographics, the lack of access, and the all-important cultural parameters impacting chronic disease. States remain hindered by a lack of critical science in the area of behavioral healthcare motivation. After all, we cannot simply throw darts at the problem of incentives and hope one scores a bull's-eye.

Medicaid cannot ethically make a new policy in this area without evidence that incentives truly work to motivate patients to improve their health risks. The science is beginning to emerge, in a limited fashion, within the private sector. We are actually seeing remarkable and successful pilot programs within corporations that use highly-effective benefit designs to rein in costs and increase quality. These pilot programs are changing how employees participate with their employer, partnering to improve health outcomes.

The private-sector approaches to controlling escalating medical costs are transferable to the Medicaid system. To incorporate the best practices from the private sector, we may need to evolve our theory and policy around our entitlement programs. Just the word entitlement seems to suggest a culture free of incentives and motivations to improve. Understanding and deploying incentives to improve quality outcomes and reduce medical costs is in the best interest of every Medicaid patient.

Our health liberties, including the right to access public assistance programs, needs to be bought with the price of our personal responsibility. That responsibility needs to be demonstrated in our attention to our high-risk behaviors. The responsibility includes avoiding chronic diseases. Without incentives to avoid and treat these diseases, we as patients are left with few options to help us modify our high-risk behaviors. Perhaps it is time to enshrine in our public health policy the fact that medical costs can be controlled by implementing appropriate incentives proven to change patient behavior.

Chapter 6
Reference List

Budget Highlights: 2007-09 Recommended Budget; The North Carolina State Budget Summary of Recommendations 2007-2009. DT McCoy. 2007.

News Release: Medicaid Spending Projected to Rise Much Faster Than the Economy. U.S. Department of Health & Human Services, 2008.

Medicaid Medical Management: A Complex Challenge for States. The Deloitte Center for Health Solutions, Deloitte Development LLC, 2011.

Proposals Approved by the NYS Medicaid Redesign Team Feb 24, 2011. New York State, 2011.

Texas State Government General Revenue Funding for Medicaid. Texas Hospital Association, 2011.

Total State Expenditures Per Capita, SFY 2007. The Henry J. Kaiser Family Foundation, 2011.

United States: Medicare Beneficiaries as a Percent of Total Population, 2010. The Henry J. Kaiser Family Foundation, 2011.

Adamy, J. Arizona Proposes Medicaid Fat Fee. 2011.

Buescher, P, J. T. Whitmire, and B Pullen-Smith. SCHS Studies: Medical Care Costs for Diabetes Associated with Health Disparities Among Adults Enrolled in Medicaid in North Carolina. North Carolina Department of Health and Human Services, 2011.

Chamberlain, J and J DeMorey. Diet and Exercise Delay Diabetes and Normalize Blood Glucose. U.S. Department of Health and Human Services, 2011.

Frieden, TR. Centers for Disease Control and Prevention: Morbidity and Mortality Weekly Report. U.S. Department of Health and Human Services, 2011.

Iglehart, John K. "Medicaid at a Crossroads." New England Journal of Medicine 364.17 (2011): 1585-87.

Legal & Regulatory Affairs Staff. Reimbursement for Telehealth Services. APA Practice Organization, 2011.

Luhby, T. Rising Medcaid Costs to Blow Hole in State Budgets.Cable News Network, A Time Warner Company, 2010.

Papp, EM. U.S. Department of Transportation. U.S. Federal Motor Carrier, Safety Administration, 2011.

Plexcia, M, H Herrick, and L Chavis. "Improving Health Behaviors in an African American Community: The Charlotte Racial and Ethnic Approaches to Community Health Project." American Journal of Public Health 98.9 (2008): 1678-84.

Pomerantz, J, S Toney, and Z Hill. "Care Coaching: An Alternative Approach to Managing Comorbid Depression." Professional Case Management Volume 15 Number 3.May/June 2010 (2011): 137-42.

Williamson, DE, Miller, TM, McVay, J, and Hinds, B. Diabetes in Alabama. 1-26. 7-2-0011. Montgomery, AL, Alabama Department of Public Health. 6-15-2011.

Σ

CHAPTER 7

Medicare in Jeopardy and What to Do About It

Picture in your mind's eye the following event. We have been crowned king and queen of a powerful and prosperous country. We plan how to spend the tax revenues graciously collected from our generous citizens. Our world-class kingly advisors prepare a spending budget, and provide a plan for our review (just after we feast on our favorite flam). We are informed by our advisors that our example budget follows the spending pattern of a very rich neighboring country. Initially, we are overjoyed with the amount of money we have to spend. Our excitement quickly turns to surprise. We learn that before anything else is done we need to set aside 7 out every 10 dollars that have been collected on healthcare, defense and pensions. That leaves only 3 tax dollars out of 10 tax dollars for every other government program. In fact, to keep up with the costs of diseases facing our population we need to spend five times more on healthcare than we spend on education and transportation combined. We realize that we spend almost as much on healthcare as we do on defense. Our advisors inform us that we need to spend the same amount of our tax revenue managing our chronic diseases, as we spend on defending ourselves against every other country in the world.

More startling is that our benevolent government, in order to cover public healthcare costs, is expected to tax each family of 4 over $10,000 a year. This is on top of what a family of four pays for out of their own pocket for health insurance, or another $6,000 dollars a year. (National Health Expenditures Aggregate, Per Capita Amounts, Percent Distribution, and Average Annual Percent Growth: Selected Calendar Years 1960-2009)

Disconcertingly, we are informed that we will need to increase our tax revenues 400% to cover the increase in healthcare expenses coming from our older citizens. This just so happens to be the case with our neighboring country. Their advisors warn:

> ...fully funding the benefits promised to present and future beneficiaries... would require permanently and immediately increasing the Medicare payroll tax rate [from ~3 percent] to roughly 13.4 percent of all wages, salaries, and self-employment income. (Foertsch and Antos)

This is just to keep up with the predictable costs we know are coming our way, especially those costs associated with hospitalization.

> The HI fund [Hospital Insurance Fund for Medicare] fails the test of short-range financial adequacy, as projected assets drop below one year's projected expenditures early in 2011. The fund also continues

to fail the long-range test of close actuarial balance. *Medicare's HI Trust Fund is expected to pay out more in hospital benefits and other expenditures than it receives in income in all future years.* The projected date of HI Trust Fund exhaustion is 2024. (Status of the Social Security and Medicare Programs: A Summary of the 2011 Reports)

What our wise advisors are telling us is that we need to think seriously about how we can reduce our medical expenses, especially hospitalization. Otherwise, we run the risk of not being able to afford care to all of our citizens and threaten the quality of our care.

This chapter is about viewing, not an imaginary scenario, but one that is playing out as we speak. This is a report of our national healthcare spending trend and creating a plan to deal with a key cost driver, namely the loss of our beta cells and other assorted chronic diseases. We spend almost the same amount on defense as we do on healthcare. Defense represents 15% of our budget, while health care represents 17%. (United States Federal, State and Local Government Spending)

While defense spending may be dramatically reduced through pulling our troops out of ongoing wars around the world, the same approach cannot be applied to the healthcare spending curve. The healthcare cost drivers are firmly in high gear. Nothing deployed to date, from a government policy perspective, has made a dent in preventing the chronic diseases that are the costliest to the system.

Preventing the diseases in the first place requires all of us to change our behavior. The government recognizes that no one has the science down when it comes to changing patient behavior. (McKay Section D1) noted that the Centers for Disease Control and Prevention (CDC) awarded grants totaling over $250,000,000 to assist policy makers with validating ways to change behaviors among high risk populations (e.g. childhood obesity). Modern science brought us the microscopic understanding of infectious processes, but little or no understanding of proven initiatives designed to modify the high risk behaviors of chronic overeating and lack of adequate physical activity.

The reason this science is so important, especially for diabetes management, is that the total direct and indirect dollar costs associated with the treatment of diabetes are estimated at ~ $174,000,000,000. To put this into perspective:

- The annual direct and indirect costs associated with diabetes exceed the individual Gross National Product of 75% of the countries in the world.
- 50% of the US states have economies that are smaller than $174 billion. The annual estimated costs associated with treating diabetes exceed the total gross domestic product of the state of Alabama.

Please turn the page to review the estimated diabetes costs in the United States as of 2007.

Chapter 7
Table 1

Table Estimated Diabetes Costs in the United States, 2007

Total costs — direct and indirect	$174 billion
Direct medical costs	$116 billion — after adjusting for population age and sex differences, average medical expenditures among people with diagnosed diabetes were 2.3 times higher than what expenditures would be in the absence of diabetes
Indirect costs	$58 billion — disability, work loss, premature mortality

(Estimated Diabetes Costs in the United States, 2007)

Most striking is that the vast majority of the costs associated with diabetes are preventable. One author notes:

High [hospital] admission rates for these potentially preventable conditions may indicate a need for improvements in access to ambulatory care and in the quality of care provided, <u>as well as in patient adoption of healthy lifestyles and active self-management of chronic conditions.</u> Thus, reducing the frequency of potentially preventable hospitalizations would be an effective strategy for lowering costs while improving quality of care and patient outcomes. Hospitalization rates for potentially preventable conditions were highest among residents in poorer communities but lowest among residents from wealthier communities. This disparity was particularly evident for diabetes without complications, <u>where the admission rate in the poorest communities was more than 400 percent higher than the rate in the wealthiest communities.</u> [emphasis added] (Jiang, Russo, and Barrett)

To prove the point that diabetes hospital costs can be controlled, a beautifully designed study was conducted within our Medicare population to see if somehow a dent could be made in the trajectory of hospital costs. Below is the study summary.

<u>Bright spot</u>

As reported in the *American Journal of Managed Care*, (Rosenzweig et al. 157-62), patients with diabetes and heart disease (most likely caused by their diabetes), and those patients with very high hospitalization rates were enrolled in this study. These patients were given telephonic access to health care providers that discussed their disease with them and provided suggests on ways to manage their medication, meals, and activity levels with the primary goal of keeping them in healthy balance. Their hospital admission rates and emergency room visit rates, along with their relative disease control, were then compared to those in a group that was used as a benchmark. This benchmark group did not have the wonderful benefit of the phone discussions with a healthcare professional around what was working, and what was not working, in their personal healthcare.

The results of this study are striking. The treated group members, those diabetes patients with heart disease that had a regularly scheduled phone call to assess how they were doing, were admitted to the hospital far less often than those patients who were not followed closely by phone. In fact, on average, these patients had costs $5,000 a year less than those patients who were without the phone support. This amount of money could really add up, especially considering the hundreds of thousands of patients that have similar diabetes related conditions. Even more gratifying for the researchers were the study findings that the clinical lab values for the treatment group improved, indicating that the treatment group actually improved their health status.

From this important study, we conclude that with the right interventions, and the right incentives, much of the hospital and treatment costs for the sickest patients with diabetes are reducible. This is a proven strategy to help win back our financial condition, as it relates to the substantial strain on our nation's healthcare resources. But many senior patients may simply say, "To heck with this phone call stuff, just leave me alone and let me take care of myself." Although, we can all applaud the self-assured and self-reliant nature of these comments, the facts indicate that our senior citizens are not aware of the cost differences between what they pay into the Medicare system through their taxes, verses what their medical costs total, at the end their lives.

To examine this carefully consider the example of David and Beth. Both David and Beth are the same age. They are the beginning wave of the baby boomer generation - a generation where it was not too uncommon for both of the husband and wife to work and have careers. According to *The National Review's* estimate, David and Beth, on average, over the course of their careers, contributed through the Medicare payroll tax approximately $45,000 dollars each, or nearly $90,000 combined. Quite a sizable sum, a sum they should be quite proud of in terms of contributing to their self-sufficiency. This is a contribution that no other generation, in the history of the United States, has created for their retirement medical care. However, expert actuarial statisticians and scientists estimate, on average, David and Beth will cost, as a couple, nearly three times that amount, before they go on to the great beyond, or nearly $360,000 total. This means that on average all of us are contributing only a third of what is needed to cover our medical expenses in retirement! Or, put another way, our medical costs will, on average, be three times greater than the amount of taxes we are now paying into Medicare. (De Rugy)

Fortunately for us there is a simple (not easy) solution for us all to cover this expenditure gap. We simply need to roughly quadruple the taxes we pay to Medicare, from 3 percent to 12-13% of our gross income. That is simple enough, just add an additional 10% tax to all of our income, so we pay for our medical care in the future and do not bankrupt the country. For some reason (ha ha) this is not politically expedient, and any politician purporting this to be part of a party platform is guaranteed defeat.

The only solution presented to date is to just borrow our way out, and thank the younger generation for the nice ride. Most experts believe we really cannot afford this strategy. A straight forward strategy would be to develop educational information that assists us in staying healthy in our old age. The federal government expertly accomplished this, as exemplified by the web site in this reference. (Young At Heart: Tips for Older Adults)

There is a consensus among government experts highlighting the healthy behaviors of older Americans. These behaviors are carefully examined in the areas of sleep, activity, nutrition, and sociality. Faithfully following guidelines established by the government task force may reduce obesity, diabetes, heart disease, cancer, and stroke. Followed consistently, these habits of healthy living can mitigate mental illnesses such as depression. Examining healthy lifestyles of the elderly brings to the forefront vital information that for many decades was underestimated in terms of its value and importance to seniors. To showcase this information, we will look at the life of Thelma, a 69 year old widowed Chicago suburb senior citizen. Walking through Thelma's daily routine gives us the perfect glimpse into the picture of healthy living for a senior citizen receiving Medicare.

Thelma loves her breakfast. She gave up soul food long ago after her husband of thirty years, Gus, died tragically of heart disease at 59 years of age. Thelma vowed that she would not let that happen to her because she wanted so desperately to participate in her grandchildren's lives for the long run. Thelma enjoys cooking cracked wheat for breakfast and adds fresh fruit and whole grain toast, and a glass of non-fat milk for her morning time meal. She is religious about eating breakfast as she found it helps her with her energy level for the balance of the day. It also aids by reducing her urge to snack on junk food. What makes breakfast even more meaningful for Thelma is that usually one of her grandchildren will call to check in with her and see that she has everything she needs.

After eating, Thelma works around the house, keeping her three-bedroom, two bath home neat and tidy. She then either works in the yard or goes for a nice hour-long walk with her pet poodle, Max. She loves the walk with Max because she meets and greets the neighbors and checks in with how they are doing. In fact, it was during one of her walks that she met Betty. Betty encouraged Thelma to volunteer three times a week for two hours at the local community hospital. She provides service at an information kiosk and helps visitors locate their loved ones. The friends at the hospital have meant a lot to her because they go out for lunch once a month and always have a good time.

Returning home from volunteering, Thelma prepares a grocery shopping list which includes certain items. Because she is on a fixed income, she must watch what she buys in order to maximize the nutrition she needs for her active lifestyle. At the top of her list are whole grains, vegetables (especially leafy, green veggies like spinach), brown rice, beans, and fruit. She makes a delicious, flavorful bean soup. Also, on her list are dairy items, such as low-fat milk, yogurt and cheese. She buys meat sparingly and usually finds the lean cuts of beef, chicken and turkey. Fish is a favorite. She learned from her friends at the hospital how to cook fish in a way that does not require a lot of butter. She also buys an assortment of dried fruits and nuts for her snack food.

Shortly before Gus's untimely death, Thelma learned to cook with recipes using fresh vegetables. She never realized how important avoiding fatty, salty, and sugary foods was until her doctor told Gus that his unhealthy eating was affecting his quality of life. Since she lost Gus at such an early age, Thelma researched and educated herself on healthy food principles and revised how she approached her eating and physical activity.

Thelma gives us a realistic glimpse of a healthy, ideal lifestyle for a senior citizen. This picture includes:

Ideal Lifestyle for a Senior Citizen

- High social contact with family, friends, neighbors, or other loved ones
- Very nutritious food shopping and meal preparation
- Little if any sweets, fatty foods or salty foods
- Daily exercise or activity
- Continued education
- Volunteerism
- Medically directed weight loss and ideal weight maintenance
- Plenty of water
- Good sleep

In the above example, Thelma has many life experiences and motivators that assist in maintaining a healthy lifestyle, including:

- Loving family, friends, neighbors and associates
- Loss of a loved one due in part to poor nutrition and inappropriate activity levels
- Access to medical care and good medical information
- A loving pet needing attention – go Max!

Senior citizens, like all of us, may need additional incentives to either motivate healthy behavior, or at the least encourage maintenance of good habits. Perhaps we can examine one motivational tactic that may be an appropriate and positive force in Thelma's life as well.

MediGap Insurance Copay Differential

MediGap insurance is purchased independently from Medicare and covers out-of-pocket expenses not included in the standard benefit. This extra insurance is of great benefit to those Medicare patients who may have developed a chronic medical condition needing frequent physician visits or hospitalizations. This add-on insurance could be the source of a potential incentive to curb overall Medicare costs. To increase the availability of this benefit, consider the following example: suppose new Medicare patients automatically qualified for reduced monthly copays for a MediGap insurance plan of their choosing if they are able to qualify based on their healthy weight, and as a non-smoker.

This concept alone, offering a greatly discounted valuable insurance, would be a clear motivation for all of us approaching retirement. Each year prior to retirement, an assessment of our weight and smoking status could be conducted to confirm our probable eligibility for this added value Medicare product. Knowing that we qualified would put this benefit into the incentive category of financial security and therefore would enact the forceful psychological factors that suggest we change our behavior in order to avoid possible loss of that security. Perhaps we would change our behavior to ensure we are healthy and remain non-smokers as we enter retirement.

If one percent of the potential Medicare population avoided diabetes, it would save hundreds of millions of dollars a year. If a portion of the Medicare benefit depended on avoiding preventable obesity and diabetes (by simply maintaining a healthy weight), we would be motivated to do cartwheels to avoid losing this part of our benefits. In the process, we would save Medicare billions of dollars.

Guaranteed: we all are going to die and most of us *will* take a lot with us when we do.

This discussion is sticky and some may want to call it stinky. The subject pertains to our eventuality—the final event of our life—our own death.   In discussing this emotional concept, we may need to understand what our medical expenses may look like shortly before we "go toward the light". We need to also avoid the political hyperbole noted in the current healthcare reform debate that foreshadows a government bureaucracy overseeing who lives and who dies. Death panel discussions are for the faint of heart politicians who are unable to propose real reform legislation designed to contain health care costs.

As it turns out, it is far more important to examine where we die than when and how we die. The problem with where we die is that we eventually end up in the hospital with tubes running helter-skelter to our life support systems, versus at home holding the hand of our loved ones. Here is the real deal.

One out every 3 dollars spent on health care is spent in the last year of our lives—primarily from hospital stays. 27 percent, or one out of every 4 dollars, of all Medicare expenses, fall into this category. Of the 27 percent, three quarters of it occurs in the last month of life. Dying in the hospital is a drain on our healthcare system and a drain on household finances. The irony is that the vast majority of us want to die at home, while at the same time, the vast majority of us take no steps to ensure that this happens. What makes this situation even more painful (no pun intended), is that all of the high-intensity care and procedures thrown at us as we are dying really end up being of no value in relation to what we need the most: less pain and an easy transition. Chillingly, reported in the prestigious medical journal, *Archives of Internal Medicine,* is this finding: "Despite this intensive resource use, studies suggest that when lifesaving treatments are unsuccessful, hospitalized patients often die with distressing symptoms." In other words, everyone is trying so hard to save our life that no one is doing the basics necessary to ease our pain and suffering. We end up dying anyway, at great cost to the system, to the tune of hundreds of millions of dollars. In actual fact, an end-of-life hospital stay for a patient with diabetes can easily reach $50,000. (End-of-Life Care Has 'Room for Improvement'), (Harding)

We may well ask, "But, why not die in the hospital; it is no skin off my nose, and by the way, this is one bill I am never going to see." That's right, the most expensive bill any of us will ever have will not even be seen by those who incur it. We are long gone, and doing the quick step in front of our Maker before the ink on that bill even dries. Peter, at the pearly gates, is not checking to see if we paid for the defibulator.

So here we are together again, realizing that it is a lack of incentives in our system that is causing it to explode with costs. Perhaps we can change the system so that two things occur. Firstly, we/the government must incentivize every Medicare recipient to have an advanced directive on file.

Secondly, earlier in their end-of-life care, every chronic disease Medicare patient needs to be evaluated for hospice care.

Advanced Directive

What is an advanced directive? A clear answer is provided by the National Library of Medicine and the National Institutes of Health:

Advance directives are legal documents that allow you to convey your decisions about end-of-life care ahead of time. They provide a way for you to communicate your wishes to family, friends and health care professionals, and to avoid confusion later on.

A living will tells how you feel about care intended to sustain life. You can accept or refuse medical care. There are many issues to address, including:

- The use of dialysis and breathing machines
- If you want to be resuscitated if breathing or heartbeat stops
- Tube feeding
- Organ or tissue donation

Continuing:

A durable power of attorney for health care is a document that names your health care proxy. Your proxy is someone you trust to make health decisions if you are unable to do so. (Advance Directives)

To help reduce the incredible financial pressures facing our healthcare system, all Medicare patients need to 1) assign a proxy with power of attorney over medical decisions and 2) specify end of life care. As an incentive to do so, if Medicare patients refuse to place this document on file with Medicare, a premium differential might be applied that approximates $36,000. This amount could be annualized over the average life span of a senior citizen entering Medicare—or approximately 18 years, or $2,000 dollars a year—and cancelled once the document is on file. This incentive is motivating and feasible, and does not raise costs to the government. (Life table for the total population: United States, 2005)

These documents can be easily created and completed online, or individualized and uploaded–all at no expense to the individual. The important point is that no one is forced to select any particular option for end-of-life treatment. In other words, we are not mandated to select "no resuscitation" or "organ donation". Once the filing of the form is made mandatory, with a financial incentive aligned to it, the vast majority of Medicare patients will complete an advanced directive. Just as soon as these come on-line, an immediate financial benefit will occur because 5% of the Medicare population passes away every year. It is this 5% that in the last month of their lives consume 20% of all Medicare costs.

What percentage of US adults have advanced directives and power of attorney proxies? A 2008 HHS report to Congress estimated that only 18% to 36% of [all] Americans had completed an advance directive. (Lexer, Kendall, and Kessler)

The secret to the success of this end-of-life process is to ensure a universal ability to centrally access the documents.

This access enables the simultaneous viewing by all healthcare workers and family members, and facilitates the handling of unexpected emergencies resulting in end-of-life situations. In many end-of-life instances, family members are conflicted with differences of opinions as to how to proceed. In order to be safe, they take the side of aggressive intervention. In reality, the odds are that the patient does not want any heroics performed to save their life, especially if medical professions determine that death is certain, and cannot be prevented by extraordinary intervention.

Consider this next Medicare incentive. It is a simple process that will speed the use of advanced directives. It is to reimburse nurses or physicians for the time it takes to discuss advance directives to Medicare patients. "A 90-minute meeting that will decide on the use of $100,000 of potential healthcare resources will be reimbursed on the order of $100 or less. It's the substantial undervaluing of this activity that is such an issue." (Kane)

We have so many excellent incentives built into the healthcare system to save lives (doctors and hospitals get paid for all procedures), but few that incentivize regarding how to close our lives gracefully, especially when the end is inevitable. Enabling our concerned healthcare providers, especially our doctors, with remuneration so they can simply guide us through the basic steps of completing and filing an advance directive may be an incredibly simple, yet powerful, way to have us responsibly prepared for the inevitable.

One unnecessary hospitalization at the end of a life could save an average of $50,000 for patients with chronic diseases like diabetes. Perhaps we can make it financially important to those who are in a position to have the discussion, based on the medical facts and history of the Medicare patient, in an environment where family members or proxies can attend and participate. Answering the inevitable questions and concerns of all of us in this situation takes a lot of time and effort, and yet the physician's time is not even considered as a possible solution to the underuse of advanced directives.

The lack of physician reimbursement can be remedied quite easily by establishing a billing code for the consultation. Perhaps the physician is paid once the advanced directive paperwork is officially registered with Medicare, as we suggested previously. Synergizing with providers on this issue will bring immediate financial savings to the system. In the not-so-distant past, when Medicare was well funded, these types of incentives were unnecessary, but due to medical advancements and a tremendous increase in baby boomer enrollment in Medicare, pilot studies emphasizing patient behavior incentives, need careful consideration. (Lubell) (Lexer, Kendall, and Kessler)

Next, we examine available healthcare market services that encourage us to remain in our homes with our loved ones as we approach our end-of-life situations. These services are contained in the wonderful program known as hospice. Hospice is end-of-life medical care usually directed at home by visiting nurses after a determination is agreed upon that end-of-life is certain in the near term. Studies confirm that hospice reduces cost while increasing the comfort of the patient. (Hospice Care Saves Money for Medicare, New Study Shows Average Savings of $2,309 per

Hospice Beneficiary) Researchers found that hospice reduced Medicare costs by an average of $2,309 per hospice patient.

Additionally, the study showed that Medicare costs would be reduced for seven out of ten hospice recipients if hospice has been used for a longer period of time.

> Given that hospice has been widely demonstrated to improve quality of life of patients and families...the Medicare program appears to have a rare situation whereby something that improves quality of life also appears to reduce costs;

This, according to the lead author Don, H. Taylor, Jr., assistant professor of public policy at Duke's Sanford Institute of Public Policy.

It is logical to ask the question, "Why don't chronically ill Medicare patients with short life-span estimates have hospice scheduled as part of their routine treatment plan?" The reasons why they do not are many, including the extreme emotionality of the topic, wherein both patients and family may be in complete denial of the pending death of their loved one. Yet, if we look deeper, we see that there is also no financial incentive to have the discussion. So, in many appropriate cases, the discussion does not occur. No one has the temerity to suggest finances should play a role in end-of-life decisions. In reality, families do have this discussion at some point. Usually, it occurs too late in the treatment plan, when the patient is hospitalized and sustained only on life support with no hope for resuscitation.

We need incentives that are thousands of dollars in value, like the advanced directives incentive above, for each

Medicare patient, and perhaps their family caregiver, that encourages them to register for hospice care prior to the actual need. From the earlier quote, we realize that most hospice care is provided too late in the end-of-life stage to have profound financial impact. If patients and family members are prepared, hospitalizations may be avoided.

Our proposed incentives for proactive hospice registration are simple. One or more of these incentives may be necessary. Below are several incentives, to name a few, that can be tied to those Medicare patients that agree to advance directives and to enter hospice rather than the hospital, once it is determined that what they are medically experiencing is terminal:

- Federal Incentives:
  - o Reduced estate probate taxes.
  - o Waive the current donut hole in the pharmacy benefit (which is modified and removed under healthcare reform). The donut hole is the point at which Medicare patients must pay the full amount for their medications.
  - o Reduced Medicare premiums, copay's, and deductibles if hospice arrangements are agreed upon by the family and are then registered in advance with Medicare.
- State Incentives:
  - o Reduce property taxes, for a minimum of six months in which hospice care is provided:
    - For the owner of the primary resident used to care for the patient.
    - For the family care giver if hospice is provided in their home.

- Corporate Incentive:
  - o Ensure job protection, or bonus, for full-time family member caregivers.
  - o Insurance incentive (i.e. disability insurance): a policy that permits the caregiver to receive 60% of their salary for assisting a loved one enrolled in hospice.

Without incentives for proactively engaging hospice services, there may continue to be a <u>substantial rise</u> in healthcare costs when an effort is made to maintain life, even when the short-term prognosis is terminal. So, the story around hospice is very compelling not only because it reduces overall costs, but also because it provides for a higher quality of life leading up to death (slightly ironic). To see a clear picture of how hospice works, consider the hypothetical case of Mr. Jones of Denver, Colorado.

<u>Mr. Jones</u>

Mr. Jones, age 81, had smoked for 5 decades and was not surprised when his doctor found a cancerous mass on his lungs that was determined inoperable due to its location, extra-large size, and type. When asked by Mr. Jones, his doctor gave him an estimate of 18 months to live. The physician suggested there was a very small chance that chemotherapy and radiation may extend his life a few months, and that both were a potential option for him to consider. Undergoing these treatments would be extremely uncomfortable, and would dramatically affect his quality of life. The doctor encouraged Mr. Jones to discuss his health status and treatment options with his family. If he was comfortable doing so, he could return in a week to map out his care for the duration of his life. The physician also encouraged Mr. Jones to look into advance directives, living wills, and to read up on hospice care.

Breaking his news to his family was difficult. Mr. Jones' wife had passed away 2 years prior in an automobile accident, so he was left with his immediate family consisting of two sons and a daughter. Both a son and daughter lived within driving distance of his home. He asked them to come over to his home and discuss his prognosis with him. Fortunately, his daughter was a lawyer specializing in family law, and his son owned his own business that enabled him to set his own schedule. After laying out all of the options with his family, he decided the best course of action for himself was to stay at home as long as possible, and when he became incapacitated, he would ask for hospice care to be delivered through his Medicare benefit while he stayed with his son. The family was in full agreement.

In discussing his treatment course with his physician, Mr. Jones mentioned his primary concern was pain, as well as his personal care needs towards the end of his life while at his son's home. To handle both of his real concerns, the physician confirmed he could prescribe for him palliative care, including the services of a hospice team when the time came. The physician assured him that he was making a sound choice to proceed in this direction, and that palliative care included pain management that was self-directed. Mr. Jones had the comfort of knowing that if pain was too severe, he, with the help of his doctor, could up the dose of pain medicine, or change the pain medicine to one that would make his life comfortable. Pain was his greatest fear.

Mr. Jones second-greatest fear was personal grooming issues. For this, he was very grateful that his son stepped up to offer supportive care. This helped him manage his concerns around his bathroom and dressing needs. Included in hospice care would be a visiting nurse to help with his entire medical issues and treatment plan, including pain management, and, if it came to it, catheter management. The son agreed to train himself on this issue in order to be fully competent when the time came.

Mr. Jones' knowledgeable daughter helped him create a living will that included an advanced health directive with restrictions on resuscitation and feeding tubes. His daughter was given power of attorney and could act as proxy for all medical emergencies, should he not be competent to make decisions. Mr. Jones was adamant that he wanted to be at his son's home when he passed, hopefully surrounded by his children and their spouses. His family was in accordance with his wishes, and was prepared for the eventuality of his passing. They all understood that, towards the end, when their father finally took a turn for the worst, that they would work through the issues to ensure that he was not in pain, and that he could remain at home. Although emotionally and physically difficult for all of them, they were on the same page.

As it turned out, things progressed similarly to how the doctor had originally explained. The doctor's input was the stimulus nucleus for Mr. Jones to take action on his end-of-life planning, including hospice care, advance directives, and a living will. When the time came for Mr. Jones to need palliative care, including pain management, the doctor prescribed high doses of a pain killer. As his time came to a close, Mr. Jones moved in with his loving son who proceeded to do his very best to serve him. In very difficult circumstances, a visiting nurse trained in hospice care was able to make additional visits and provide extra support and compassion to the family. Mr. Jones passed away in his sleep some fourteen months after his diagnosis.

The importance of this case study is multifaceted. Note that the family was able to make advance preparations, with the support of each other and Mr. Jones' physician. Not all of us will be so fortunate. Nor will we all be so lucky as to have loving children by our side to take care of us at the very end. Nonetheless, there are a vast number of Medicare patients and their families that do fall into a similar scenario, and may be organized in advance for in the final stages of a senior parent's life. Furthermore, this care pattern is supportable by the incentives discussed in this chapter.

Mr. Jones could have already prepared an advanced directive and a living will with the help of his daughter, as we all can, depending on our finances. Perhaps, if the incentives discussed above were in place, Mr. Jones would have already prepared his advanced directives well in advance of his diagnosis. In addition, when he turned 80, the good doctor would have reinforced the same discussion on advance directives, not just because it was the right thing to do, but because he was reimbursed for his time. With the tremendous shortage of family practice physicians, time is becoming an important commodity.

Most of us have real concerns about how we will exit this life, especially in terms of our personal privacy, finances, and pain. These issues are extremely important and under-discussed in most families, and with most doctors. If we could be assured, through advanced directives and a prepared living will, that all of our needs would be met, and if we could have our loving family in full agreement, life would more likely end gracefully. The resources saved could be handed down to the next generation. Collectively, we could conservatively estimate that the Jones family saved the health care system tens of thousands of dollars, while providing the best possible quality of life for their loving father. Mr. Jones, his family, the hospice team, and the physician are examples of heroes.

The impact of these principles, implemented with powerful incentives, can correct the debt-driven healthcare budgetary problems we all face in Medicare. These principles are not new or novel, but aligning them to incentives is new. Perhaps we can support simple, straightforward common-sense incentives that encourage and motivate us to a higher level of responsibility, especially toward the end of our lives. These incentives do not require a new program, greater costs, more training, or more legislation.

Understanding the science of incentives may dramatically increase the quality of end-of-life experience for many Medicare patients. Identifying and measuring the impact of these incentives may prove to all of us how simple motivation may shift healthy behavior of the consumers, families, and providers of Medicare. Once aligned in a direction that reinforces long term efficiency and quality, these incentives will overcome the costly outcomes that are placing our nation and families in peril.

Chapter 7
Reference List

United States Federal, State and Local Government Spending. Christopher Chantrill. U.S. Government Spending.com, 2000.

Hospice Care Saves Money for Medicare, New Study Shows Average Savings of $2,309 per Hospice Beneficiary. J. Radulovic. National Hospice and Palliative Care Organization, 2007.

Young At Heart: Tips for Older Adults. Weight-control Information Network.

National Institutes of Health, 2007.

Life table for the Total Population: United States, 2005. Vol. 58, No. 10. 3-3-2010. Center for Disease Control. National Vital Statistics Reports. 7-24-2011.

National Health Expenditures Aggregate, Per Capita Amounts, Percent Distribution, and Average Annual Percent Growth: Selected Calendar Years 1960-2009. Centers for Medicare and Medicaid Services, 2011.

Advance Directives. NIH: National Cancer Institute. U.S. National Library of Medicine

National Institutes of Health, 2011.

End-of-Life Care Has 'Room for Improvement'. R. Preidt. DAILY HEALTH PULSE, 2011.

Estimated Diabetes Costs in the United States, 2007. National Diabetes Information Clearinghouse (NDIC) 11-3892. 2011. Bethesda, MD 20892–3560, U.S. Department of Health and Human Services. 7-15-2011.

Status of the Social Security and Medicare Programs: A Summary of the 2011 Reports. Social Security and Medicare Boards of Trustees. 2011.

De Rugy, V. Medicare and Social Security: What You Pay In vs. What You Will Get (Maybe). National Review Online, 2011.

Foertsch, T. and J Antos. The Economic and Fiscal Effects of Financing Medicare's Unfunded Liabilities. The Heritage Foundation, 2011.

Harding, A. End-of-life care costs continue to climb upward. Reuters, Edition U.S., 2010.

Jiang, HJ, Russo, CA, and Barrett, ML. Nationwide Frequency and Costs of Potentially Preventable Hospitalizations, 2006. Healthcare Cost and Utilization Project. Statistic Brief #72. 2011. Rockville, MD, Agency for Healthcare Research and Quality. 7-16-2011.

Kane, L. "Why such paltry reimbursement for discussing advance directives with patients? 2-4-2010. Medscape. 7-28-2011.

Lexer, S., Kendall, D., and Kessler, J. Transforming End-of-Life Care. 7-20-2009. The Third Way. 7-26-2011.

Lubell, J. End-of-life care: Advance directives have value, but some in industry cite drawbacks, too. Modern Healthcare, 2010.

McKay, B. "Out Front in the Fight on Fat." The Wall Street Journal 26 Apr. 2011.

Rosenzweig, JL, et al. "Diabetes Disease Management in Medicare Advantage Reduces Hospitalizations and Costs." The American Journal of Managed Care 16.7 (2011): 157-62.

$$\Sigma$$

CHAPTER 8

Pharmaceutical Companies: Villains or Vanquishers

Mary was calmly making her son's favorite sandwich for his school lunch—a nice, creamy peanut butter sandwich with grape jam; hmm.... yummy. Mary smiled at the idea that she was participating in a ritual that was repeated in tens of thousands of households across America. Like most Americans, Mary would be astounded to know the facts behind her homemaker's traditional lunch staple. In the US alone, there is enough peanut butter sold to make over 10,000,000,000 (ten billion) peanut butter and jelly sandwiches each year. If you were to peer behind Americans' kitchen cupboards, you would find peanut butter in nine out of every ten homes. Have you ever wondered how much we spend on the creamy or crunchy stuff? $800,000,000 a year. (Peanuts & Peanut Butter Fun Facts)

And yet, this is just peanuts. Amazingly, as a country, we have another extremely common ritual, as evidenced by the fact that <u>we spend over twice that much on insulin</u>. Pharmaceutical companies sell well over $2 billion dollars' worth of insulin each year to Americans that can no longer produce the insulin hormone in sufficient quantities to sustain their bodies' energy requirements. They inject themselves every day with this life-saving pharmaceutical product. Pharmaceutical companies produce over 100,000 gallons of insulin a year, all of which is measured to the milliliter and delivered via pump, syringe, or insulin pen device through tiny needles, directly into the soft tissue of patients with diabetes.

To ensure that their insulin product is prescribed properly by physicians, a typical pharmaceutical company may employ 1,000 sales professionals to call on doctor offices, at a total cost of over a $100,000,000. These professionals are all well-trained in diabetes, insulin, and any potential side effects that may arise from the use of their products. In fact, for every sales call that is made to a physician, a pharmaceutical company needs to budget at least $150 in salary, training and supplies. Some representatives will make five to ten calls a day, costing over $500 per person, to deliver a pharmaceutical company's primary insulin use marketing message into the doctor's office. Having sold diabetes products for over 20 years, I can share with you the dilemma we faced on a daily basis. Although we marketed the number one product in the world to assist in the management of diabetes, as representatives we never could utter the phrases, "this product offers a cure for the disease", or "this product may prevent the disease".

Consider for a moment the incredible irony of having the best product in the world, but at the same time knowing this product was only partially able to help the patients with their disease. On top of that, we understood clearly the cost of the resources that were being allocated in the fight to save the lives of these patients. Hundreds of millions of dollars a year are spent advertising, marketing, selling, and educating the medical industry about products that only manage, not cure, chronic diseases.

> It has been estimated that pharmaceutical companies spend over $6 billion a year on marketing to physicians, 80 percent of their marketing budget. This averages to over $9,000 annually per practicing physician in this country. Drug sales representatives come to the office, leave samples, lunch, pens, pads and selected articles in order to "educate" [providers] about their new products. (Haddad)

In addition, a few of the drug companies employ a field staff of registered nurses with certification as diabetes educators, to assist patients and providers with the proper use of pharmaceutical products. This is an example of pharmaceutical companies investing tens of millions of dollars in an educational activity to help patients stay on their prescribed insulin. Patients commonly stop taking insulin due to drug intolerance, financial concerns, cultural barriers, or problems adjusting to an effective dose. Some patients simply refuse to take insulin and hope a pill can control their symptoms. Millions of dollars of potential sales are lost due to lack of patient adherence, and to the problems associated with the lack of symptom-control some patients may experience.

Although these highly trained nurses are incredibly adept at managing patients and their symptoms, in the final analysis they are also unable to suggest to the patients that the products they prescribe can cure diabetes. With the lack of patient compliance with the doctors' prescribed treatment plan of losing weight and eating healthily, along with the problems of staying on a drug like insulin that may need to be injected once or more a day, patients with diabetes may not experience optimum outcomes.

"What we have here is a failure to communicate!" (1967 Movie: *Cool Hand Luke*)

We can change this unfortunate patient outcome dynamic by changing the forces that drive the behaviors of the drug company, the providers, the insurance company, and the patient. Permit me to dramatize this for us with the following futuristic example.

John

The year is 2015. John is a 45 year-old male, newly diagnosed with type 2 diabetes that was brought on by his decades of overeating and inactivity. His physician was excited to see him. The physician had just been trained on a new approach to John's situation. This training indicated that with proper incentives in place, John could dramatically increase the chances for a successful treatment outcome. To implement the treatment, John needed to make an appointment with his doctor's nurse to watch a video. The video would explain everything, and then John could meet face to face with his doctor to determine the best course of action.

John made the appointment to watch the video and was surprised to find that as a new patient with diabetes, his symptoms were potentially reversible, if he was careful to follow the treatment plan. If he could change his high-risk eating behavior, he might be able to avoid some of the serious complications of diabetes. What really struck him, however, was the need for his passionate participation in the plan. He learned that he had already lost some beta cell function. This is what else he found out:

He is definitely not alone. The staggering reality is that over 1,000,000 people in the United States aged 45 to 64 are diagnosed with his condition each year. (National Diabetes Statistics, 2011: New Cases of Diagnosed Diabetes)

As an example, imagine that the federal government, faced with impending financial health care cost crisis, was compelled to determine the best course of treatment for patients just like John. They did this by conducting extensive research. What they found shocked them, and made the medical industry stand down. The video showed John that comparative effectiveness research, conducted with 10,000 patients, determined which class of drugs had the best results in newly diagnosed patients with diabetes. It was determined that of all the drug classes, insulin (as just one possible category of drugs) was shown to be most effective. Effectiveness was determined by weight loss, glucose control in newly diagnosed patients, and overall cost to the healthcare system.

Imagine, as the video showed John, that the studies demonstrated that if a new diabetes patient faithfully followed the full treatment plan (including weight loss), within 6 months, many could eliminate the insulin and be returned to near normal blood sugar control. The secret to this medical success, the video pointed out, was neither the drug nor the doctor's prescriptions, but the changes in the patient's own behavior. But that's not all; the patients had very specific help to make those behavioral changes.

Continue to imagine that in these well-controlled studies, patients were given behavioral health incentives, and that these incentives had major ramifications. Firstly, if patients chose not to change their high-risk eating and activity levels their insurance rates jumped significantly— from 20% to 30%. Their copayment for insulin could possibly double to 50% of the cost of the prescription. Secondly, suppose the studies found that voluntarily noncompliant patients were, in essence, wasting their medication <u>because the quantity of what they continued to eat overwhelmed the effectiveness of the drug</u>. In an attempt to help patients, the Federal Drug Administration (FDA) might conclude that patients needed to have a substantial cost incentive, in an annual range of thousands of dollars, so they would not waste drugs. This incentive was only for patients who willingly did not follow the prescribed treatment plan. The patients had no additional costs if they followed the treatment plan. In other words, for compliant patients, the treatment was all covered by their normal insurance copayments. Not only that, their prescription costs could end after six months, because in some cases, as newly diagnosed patients, their glucose and insulin could return to near normal. Patients were highly motivated to change their behavior, especially if it meant avoiding the insulin syringe needle, greater out of pocket expenses, and the complications of diabetes.

The other vitally important prescribed assistance was a home visit by a specially trained educator that reviewed the patient's home environment for proper nutrition and activity level. This trained individual assisted in developing food purchase and preparation strategies that helped patients like John remain on a healthy diet long term. The specialist reviewed the essentials of diet in conjunction with the patient's cultural preferences and budget. The educator, where appropriate, reviewed this part of the treatment plan with all those in the household responsible for food purchasing and preparation, and who had volunteered themselves to review the healthy eating information provided. Lastly, patients agreed, in writing, with the educator that they would exercise five days a week for an hour a day, in some fashion, to the best of their abilities. For the great majority of patients, this simply meant going for a walk.

John was surprised by the results that were presented in the video. The studies showed that newly-diagnosed, young patients who enrolled in the incentive program, and successfully followed it for six months, were four to six times more likely to successfully treat their diabetes, compared to patients who did not follow the prescribed treatment plan. Non-compliant patients were less likely to succeed in controlling their diabetes, and spent a lot more of their own money trying to stay healthy.

The video went on to show that the doctor John had chosen was specifically trained and certified to treat his condition, and that his doctor closely followed the national treatment guidelines that had been developed with over 40 years of research. The physician's pay structure was revised such that if he and the patient were able to succeed with the treatment plan, the physician would be compensated doubly for his effort. John had full confidence that if he followed his physician's advice closely and carefully, he would be successful.

John could not help but wonder how a pharmaceutical company could actually help a patient go off of their drug after six months and avoid disease-related complications. What he found amused him significantly. In our futuristic example it turned out that the US government realized that for each of the 1,000,000 new diabetics diagnosed each year they would be spending $300,000 of tax-payer money to treat them throughout their life span. So, they determined to change the reimbursement paradigm for the pharmaceutical companies and physicians. They determined that it was well worth providing a billion-dollar payment each year to the pharmaceutical company whose diabetes product was determined to be the most effective in controlling the disease. This approach resulted in a great cost savings, since the best product was soon revealed through comparative trials. With incentives to support the patient's own behavior changes, prescription volume was lowered, as more newly-diagnosed patients achieved glucose control faster than before. In fact, the reduction in costs associated with prescription volume was shown to far exceed the billion-dollar annual investment provided to the company selling the best product. This program resulted in higher quality, better health outcomes, and lower costs for patients and more money in the pharmaceutical company's coffers.

Lastly, John was asked if he would consent to allow the results of his treatment to be submitted anonymously into a data bank. This would enable the government to continue to track the results from the millions of patients diagnosed over several years. This body of evidence would continue to funnel into the best medical practices in the world, and deliver the information as to which were the safest and most effective protocol, products, incentives, and physician training available to treat newly-diagnosed patients with type 2 diabetes.

No wonder John needed to see this video. It demonstrated that the best medicine and the best treatment plans in the world were now being proven in real-life trials, and that his experience, although perhaps painful, serious, and concerning, would work out just fine. If he followed his treatment plan, he would not be expected to pay any additional money. Best of all, the research showed that he had a high likelihood of being free of complications for many years to come if he simply adhered to his doctor's recommendations. He was thus truly motivated to make those changes which would ensure his continued good health.

John's 2015 scenario is not that farfetched. Most of the elements in his treatment are now on the drawing board. Some of the broader issues are part of healthcare reform. Reform may bring this kind of treatment plan to all patients facing a chronic disease.

A far-reaching issue, still not resolved, is the pricing puzzle for pharmaceutical manufacturers. Their products are only occasionally tested head-to-head with the competition in order to try to demonstrate which product is superior from a quality and overall cost perspective. Branded drugs (as opposed to generic drugs) are rarely compared against one another. Pharmaceutical companies use their talented sales forces to point out their drug's advantages with physicians. The non-comparative, non-head-to-head type of studies protect companies from showing a possible weaker result, and assists them in selling more of their product, regardless of whether or not the product is superior at reducing overall medical costs and improving the patients' quality of life.

In lieu of incentivizing pharmaceutical companies to create the best product in its class, state and federal governments and other purchasing entities, may be instituting financial dis-incentives by creating mandatory rebates and cutthroat price negotiations. To support patients like John, possible future purchasing practices may need to focus on quality outcomes and overall medical cost reductions as opposed to price. Current purchasing practices may focus too heavily on lowest-price-takes-all purchasing strategies, and may not incent companies to prove that they have the overall best product. In reality, there is usually a wide variation in important product variables, such as safety, efficacy, quality, and the overall medical costs. In addition, development costs for innovating and producing the best new products may also force a higher initial price.

To be clear, the pharmaceutical industry is very profitable. A report on the pharmaceutical industry mentions:

...the pharmaceutical industry is — and has been for years — the most profitable of all businesses in the U.S. In the annual *Fortune* 500 survey, the pharmaceutical industry topped the list of the most profitable industries, with a return of 17% on revenue. (Barlett et al.)

Excalibur Potions

To demonstrate the strain pharmaceutical company senior managements are under to develop and market a new product, we will walk into a fictitious board meeting of a large imaginary company named Excalibur Potions. The board is discussing the development plans for their newly discovered fictitious diabetes medicine with the brand name: Glucobil.

Board Meeting

Ms. Board Member: "Chairman, please explain to the board how this product, Glucobil, is going to make us money."

Chairman: "Thank you very much, Ms. Board Member. Before we examine this product in detail, let me remind you briefly where we are positioned in the industry and what reasonable expectations we have for our product. First of all, I quote from *US News* that the profits for the major health care companies are stacking up to look like this.... Notice the nice returns from our competitors below (e.g. Amgen, Johnson & Johnson, and Pfizer)."

- Amgen (biotechnology): Profit margin, 30.6 percent
- Gilead Sciences (biotechnology): 37.6 percent
- Celgene Corp. (biotechnology): 11.9 percent

- Johnson & Johnson (drug manufacturer): 20.8 percent
- Pfizer (drug manufacturer): 16.3 percent
- GlaxoSmithKline (drug manufacturer): 17.4 percent
- As a comparison, UnitedHealth Group (healthcare plans): 4.1 percent
- WellPoint (healthcare plans): 4 percent
- Aetna (healthcare plans): 3.9 percent
- MedcoHealth Solutions (healthcare services): 2.1 percent
- Express Scripts (healthcare services): 3.7 percent
- Quest Diagnostics (healthcare services): 8.7 percent
- Medtronic (medical equipment): 14.9 percent
- Baxter International (medical equipment): 17.5 percent
- Covidien (medical equipment): 12.3 percent
  (Newman)

Mr. Chairman, continuing: "To answer your direct question, consider our upside sales potential. Annual topline sales of Glucobil in 5 years are projected to be 500 million dollars. At year 5, we will still be in the negative, due to substantial investments needed to develop the compound through all of the clinical trials. Importantly, due to its chemical properties, we will need to build a new manufacturing plant to produce Glucobil. These costs are as follows:

Clinical trial programs, including all phases through FDA approval: $750 million. (Masia) For every patient we track on this product through our clinical trial network, we need to budget $20,000 dollars. (Clinical Operations: Accelerating Trials, Allocating Resources and Measuring

Performance), (Phase 3 Clinical Trial Costs Exceed $26,000 per Patient)

Cost to construct the new manufacturing plant: $250 million. The total development costs, therefore, including those sunk costs that were used to find and develop the compound, is roughly $1 billion dollars." (Amgen Pharmaceutical Manufacturing Facility, United States of America)

Board Member: "That is a huge sum. Assuming we can come up with the finances to carry the development costs, what is our profit margin, and how much will we need to sell to turn a profit?"

Chairman: "Well, we do have a nice net 50% profit margin from which to work. Please remember, though, in order to compete in this sophisticated market, we will need to expand our existing sales force by 250, at an additional annual cost of $50 million, which will have a considerable impact on profits. This is essential because the number of patients we hope to have on this product will be between 200 and 500 thousand patients at any one time.

Gaining this level of sales will require an extensive marketing and sales campaign, among the largest in the industry. Based on our sales forecast and at a 50% profit margin target after year five, Excalibur Potions will clear $250 million each year. Therefore, by year 9 or 10 we will break even and thereafter clear $200 million a year. If all goes according to plan, we will have a remaining 2 or 3 years of patent protection, producing between $400 million and $600 million dollars of profit....."

As an aside, "If all goes according to plans...." Is a very relevant comment. A real-life example of the risks pharmaceutical companies face in developing new drugs can been seen by reading the history of one of the biggest potential products ever launched in the diabetes field. It failed in the market place, even after a decade of trials and marketing effort: inhaled insulin. This FDA-approved insulin could be used by breathing it into the lungs, so patients could avoid using a needle. It was removed from the market after failing to gain acceptance. All costs for those companies that invested billions of dollars to bring this product to market, including building new manufacturing plants, was never recovered. (Dairman)

Continuing our story: Chairman: "Unfortunately, I will be retired by year 5 of Glucobil's sales cycle, and will not know if we even break even. Nonetheless, as pharmaceutical agents go, Glucobil seems like a good prospect. Long term, it may help us maintain our 15% overall company profit goal, which is similar to the industry standard, and is the net profit margin our shareholders expect us to earn. From our knowledge to date, we conclude that Glucobil has substantial downstream profit potential. Excalibur Potions must move quickly, because the patent on Glucobil expires in year 7 from launch date. Accordingly, we lose downstream profitable years if we delay implementing our plans, as there will be, no doubt, the launch of numerous generic competitors immediately after Glucobil's patent expires."

From this vignette, we learn of the incredible risk that drug development carries, and the dynamic pressure on pharmaceutical companies to remain profitable. They carry the burden of massive development costs, unpredictable returns, and shortened patent life due to generic competition and lengthened clinical trial requirements. Also, from our vignette, we see that in order to recoup development and marketing costs, pharmaceutical companies must have strong year-over-year recurring sales which show a net profit for the drug. Historically, most pharmaceutical companies have been able to produce these results. Over time, however, most companies hit dry spells, where the generic competition is greater than their pace of new product development. Lack of innovation eventually drives companies into a merger situation. This boom-and-bust scenario is all too familiar for pharmaceutical executives who have seen this cycle repeat itself often.

Boom-and-bust—sounds like gold rush times and the Wild, Wild West at its best; where thousands of prospectors took to the hills in search of the vein of gold that would make them fabulously rich beyond their wildest dreams. That lure of wealth was a true incentive to leave behind the comforts of home, family, farming, and property to try and strike it rich. Of course, we know that only a tiny fraction of the hopeful wonderers actually were successful. The rest gave up their search in Alaska, Nevada, or California and returned home. The gold rush analogy relates to the boom-and-bust efforts of drug companies, and is a telling story. It shows that with a high enough potential reward, a stampede of entrepreneurs will enter the market, risking their own capital in pursuit of the prize.

Without a huge potential return on effort, no research will be conducted on a project that requires a substantial investment. To encourage the risk-takers in our economy to use their resources to uncover the solutions for chronic diseases, there must be a pot at the end, of a billion dollars or more. And so it is that only a handful of companies in the world can put up sufficient capital to go after that prize. There is another option.

The Federal Government, because it stands to save billions of dollars on effective, proven treatments, can mitigate and incentivize the risk. After all, it is the bill-payer of 50% of America's medical costs. So, we ask, what is the government doing about drug research and disease cure and treatment? How is it involved anyway, and how can we accelerate the discovery of cures, not just treatments? (The Congress of the United States)

Historically, the federal government spends about 25 billion dollars on drug research and approves approximately 10 to 20 novel new compounds a year. The private sector spends around 45 billion dollars on drug research for a combined total, between government and private industry, of $70 billion dollars. Still, only 10-20 new therapeutic compounds a year are approved across all disease states. Ninety percent of these drugs do not cure the conditions for which they are targeted. As a result, perhaps one drug a year is approved that actually cures a disease and these drugs are usually in the class of new antibiotics or vaccines. Producing one drug a year out of 70 billion dollars of research investment creates one cure for one infectious disease—that is the end result of our return on investment in pharmaceutical research. The other products may be fine additions to our choices of treatment, but they also continue to escalate our expenses, as they represent further treatment options, not permanent solutions.

Let us assume all of the drug research money spent was in one pot which includes both the government and private company research dollars. If we take the 10 to 20 new drugs approved each year, and divide it into the total spent on research between government and private industry, we find that we spend between $3 billion and $7 billion dollars a year for each new novel drug approved by the FDA. Keep this figure in mind as we move forward to examine our national priorities spent on basic disease research, brought to you again by the federal government and the affiliated National Institutes of Health (NIH).

Here is what the NIH is all about, in their own words. (About NIH: NIH Budget)

> The NIH invests a total of over $31.2 billion annually in medical research for the American people. More than 80% of the this funding is awarded through almost 50,000 competitive grants to more than 325,000 researchers at over 3,000 universities, medical schools, and other research institutions in every state and around the world. About 10% of the NIH's budget supports projects conducted by nearly 6,000 scientists in its own laboratories, most of which are on the NIH campus in Bethesda, Maryland.

Taking a closer look at the NIH, we can understand the spending priorities.

Disease	millions	Percentage
Clinical Research	10707	7.71%
Genetics	7470	5.38%
Prevention	5981	4.31%
Cancer	5823	4.19%
Biotechnology	5675	4.09%

Neurosciences	5513	3.97%
Infectious Diseases	3888	2.80%
Brain Disorders	3845	2.77%
Women's Health 5/	3689	2.66%
Behavioral and Social Science	3525	2.54%
Clinical Trials	3282	2.36%
Pediatric	3282	2.36%
Bioengineering	3162	2.28%
HIV/AIDS 6/ 12/	3086	2.22%
Health Disparities 5/	2726	1.96%
Minority Health 5/	2525	1.82%
Aging	2517	1.81%
Mental Health	2246	1.62%
Cardiovascular	2143	1.54%
Emerging Infectious Diseases	2117	1.52%
Human Genome	1903	1.37%

As noted, across all disease states, the National Institutes of Health budgets less than five percent of its funding for prevention studies. Broadly and generally speaking, prevention studies are in the minority, and few, if any, studies examine the extent to which financial incentives change health behaviors. How could they? There is too much to know about the disease state itself for NIH scientists and grantees to spend the time and resources to do the intensive research necessary to understand preventive behavior strategies that improve compliance with treatment plans. With their 30 billion plus dollars, the NIH is involved in researching the disease: transmission routes, genetic origins, molecular origins, diagnosis, and treatments.

We as tax payers need to examine how to stop preventable diseases in their tracks through behavioral interventions and incentives. Cures are simply not forthcoming. Cures are found by preventing the disease in the first place—as with vaccines. The NIH may find it useful to concentrate on finding the incentives that drive behavioral change that can cure and prevent disease. If scientists develop the evidence for the best behavior modification incentive, there might be a greater return on research dollars. Perhaps the NIH needs to partner with their industry colleagues in pharmaceutical companies to develop preventative strategies along with new, costly drug treatments.

Ninety percent of diabetes is preventable. Is 90% of the research funding for diabetes, heart disease, or stroke (which are also disease state that are highly preventable) going to identify and test for the most powerful incentives to stop the disease? I am afraid not. In fact, if you added up the funding for diabetes, heart disease and stroke you will find nearly 10% of the budget is going for research in these disease areas. Potentially, this means billions of dollars. And yet, in examining just one of these areas— cardiovascular disease—there is no mention of funding anywhere in the country for understanding behavioral incentives. Pharmaceutical companies and federal research agencies may need to consider accompanying their research with behavioral modification and lifestyle intervention programs that support patients who are dealing with chronic disease.

Solutions

Here are the top ten suggested government and drug studies that will identify the key motivational incentives which could turn us all into compliant patients and give us the ability to reduce our waistlines for good.

Changing employee behavior, potential landmark studies

Studies – finding answers by finally asking the most impactful questions:

1. Health insurance study:

What healthcare insurance benefit design is most effective in motivating at-risk patients and their at-risk dependents in reducing their health risk factors? Results could be measured by adherence to their physician-prescribed treatment plan and overall medical costs.

2. Provider Network study:

Discover which provider network in the country is most effective in reducing medical costs and improving patient satisfaction through patient compliance to a provider's prescribed treatment plan. Provider networks could measure patient satisfaction and reduced overall medical expenses.

3. Wellness program disease management study:

Determine which corporate wellness programs and disease-management programs are the most effective in reducing risky health behaviors as evidenced by a reduction in medical costs and absenteeism. Analyze the core incentive components of the study that cause such programs to be effective.

4. Medicaid incentive study:

Once it is shown that patients have been reasonably supported by culturally relevant education and training, study ethical Medicaid incentives by allowing all states to test the effectiveness of stringent financial incentives for supporting patients in their effort to follow their provider's treatment plan.

5. Medicare Incentive study:

Establish a Medicare waiver that supports a study to determine which incentives are powerful enough to encourage 1) obesity avoidance and 2) proactive end-of-life decisions, including avoiding unnecessary interventions and unnecessary hospitalizations. Include physician compensation studies to determine appropriate levels of reimbursement for their time discussing end of life options with patients and their families. Study and implement the findings of an automatic end-of-life enrollment process for all Medicare beneficiaries. Include in the study the financial and quality-of-life impact of a substantial one-time tax credit for all Medicare beneficiaries who complete end of life care enrollment processes.

6. Drug studies completed with wellness arm:

Require all new drug studies regarding chronic diseases to include an additional arm of the study with a control and treatment group which completes a wellness program. Study the effectiveness of the drug, both with and without a wellness intervention. Provide pharmaceutical companies with a process to trademark, patent, and license a proven effective wellness program that can be sold as a stand-alone product or offered as part of the prescription for the product.

7. America's Healthiest Schools Study:

Determine which schools have the healthiest students by standardized testing. Determine the causative variables and study their relative effectiveness and portability.

8. Legal Framework for Healthy Behavior Incentives Study:

Establish the legal framework from which healthy behavior incentives are made available for recipients of public health resources.

9. Legal Framework for Insurance Reforms which include Financial Incentives studies:

Study design to include the legal precedent supporting insurance reform, in order that insurance benefit designs can readily incorporate financial incentives to support patients in avoiding and treating preventable chronic diseases.

10. Personal Income Tax Relief for Avoiding Obesity:

Study and establish the legal framework for instituting a personal income tax incentive which provides a deduction to all > 21-year-old taxpayers that are in a non-obese weight category as certified by a licensed health care provider.

The list of studies could go on and on. Especially if the billions of dollars used to research diseases could be directed to finding the incentives needed for us to change our behaviors and avoid diabetes.

Congress needs to position pharmaceutical companies, state and federal governments, private corporations, and citizen groups with incentives and directives in order to perform this valuable research. Every diabetes case prevented saves $300,000 in future medical costs over the lifetime of the patient. Federal and state grant activities aimed at preventable diseases need, as a first priority, to focus their resources on evaluating the incentives that are needed to help patients adhere to a treatment plan, and remain compliant with their prescribed medications, nutrition, and activity levels.

Give big Pharma a big carrot. Take a billion dollars from the diabetes and prevention fund, find which drugs are most effective, and which wellness programs are succeeding in reducing health care costs by curbing obesity and diabetes.

Corporations can drive this activity faster than the state and local governments. Here are effective ways to do so, with little or no additional costs to the company's bottom line.

1. Establish a culture of health and wellness at the workplace.

2. Reward and incentivize healthy behaviors beyond better ergonomics and work safety reviews.

3. Create the health culture within the employee productivity review process by establishing the fact that healthy employees who are avoiding preventable diseases are more productive, and therefore need to be compensated accordingly.

4. Review the health benefit design and take time to determine which products and services provide proof of a decrease in healthcare costs.

5. Incent employees by establishing lower copays for access to these medications and services.

6. Incentivize pharmaceutical companies with enhanced positioning of their products on the approved drug list, either by reducing rebates and giving preferred

positioning, or providing employees with free education regarding the medication or service.

7. Corporations could incentivize their health insurance provider (in a confidential and secure fashion), and their elected pharmacy benefits manager (in a blinded fashion) to conduct productivity analysis to determine which employees with any given preventable chronic disease demonstrate less absenteeism, higher productivity and lower medical costs.

8. As positive causality is established, these products and services can enjoy increased recognition and support through incentivizing a lower cost to the employee.

9. The Institute for Health and Productivity (IHPM.org) can assist in conducting and publishing the results of these studies. The findings of these studies can assist all stakeholders in purchasing and educational investment decisions.

Premium Educational Programs and the Pharmaceutical Industry

Where can we find the money to sponsor such studies? Pharmaceutical and biotechnology companies spent over two billion dollars a year on professional education for providers in much of the previous decade. This education met the criteria for continuing education for physicians, nurses, and pharmacists (CME or CE). The industry has implemented changes, but as of 2004, when the following was reported, it provided a historic view into incentives and how pharmaceutical companies felt that education could help market their products. (Fugh-Berman and Batt 412-15)

...more than $2 billion was spent on CME; pharmaceutical manufacturers paid for more than half of that sum. Firms that manufacture FDA-regulated products (primarily pharmaceuticals) provided three-quarters (74.7 percent) of the income of medical education and communication companies (MECCs). CME provided by medical schools is almost equally reliant on the pharmaceutical industry, which provides almost two-thirds (63.8 percent) of CME income to medical schools.

Much has changed over the ensuing years, but it may be time to rethink how CME education is underwritten. It is imperative for medical device and drug manufactures to not just deliver their product to market, but to deliver it relevant to a system of care that reduces costs, increases quality, and provides enhanced patient engagement, compliance, and proven outcomes. Perhaps to meet the qualification for CME, companies providing education must have this data on file, published, or peer reviewed before CME-granting entities designate their education as meeting the standards for such high distinction. This data and education needs to contain research on which behavioral incentives can assist patients with disease prevention. Surely some of the billions deployed for education can be earmarked for this incredibly important service to our patient and medical education community.

Chapter Summary

Pharmaceutical companies have revolutionized the treatment of chronic diseases with breakthrough therapies in blood pressure control and diabetes. The best of these therapies have extended lives, increased the quality of life, and truly enhanced the productivity of many patients. The United States stands apart as the greatest source of new product development, and is a primary means of supplying superior science and technology in the area of drug development to the entire world. As medical costs continue to explode, it becomes apparent that we need to maximize our return on product marketing such that resources are deployed to further our understanding of not only the safety and efficacy of products, but of the overall cost-effectiveness of the product or service.

To accomplish this mission, pharmaceutical companies need new market incentives through new FDA legislation and/or public and private payers requiring outcome studies demonstrating superior results to current therapy. These outcome studies need to include the examination of incentives that help patients avoid the disease and potential complications. The economic return, large enough to change this research direction, needs to account for the tremendous capital investments made by most innovative pharmaceutical firms.

Incentives for these companies could provide an enhanced return through faster market share development, an extended patent life, or preferred placement on drug lists. Manufactures will be motivated by these new incentives, and incorporate them as part of their drug development costs, especially if the incentives are in place to foster faster, longer, and greater market access. These incentives will produce a win for consumers, pharmaceutical companies and the payers of healthcare.

As consumers, we can bend the healthcare cost curve that is facing all of us by doing a couple of things. Firstly, we can all stay closely compliant to our prescribed treatment plan. This means seeing the doctor regularly, taking our prescribed medicine, watching carefully what we eat, and participating in the right level of activity to match our abilities and health status. We can participate fully in our employer-sponsored wellness and disease-management programs. We can actively participate in our own disease prevention by changing our culture to include financial incentives and motivations for us to stay healthy.

Secondly, as policy makers, we can incentivize pharmaceutical companies by providing greater reimbursement and patient access to proven effective medications. We can reward pharmaceutical companies for products and lifestyle interventions that document a reduction in disease costs, overall medical costs, and improved quality of life. We can extend patent life and greater patient access for products that also offer patient and provider education that are proven to be the most effective in their class at improving quality of life and reducing total medical costs.

Thirdly, we need to properly align and incentivize our 70 billion dollar medical product research priorities, so that the focus is shifted to patient behaviors, the root cause of most preventable diseases. Pharmaceutical company resources can vanquish such diseases by attaching lifestyle intervention research to all new product development. *Dianomics* suggests that economic incentives, properly aligned towards disease prevention, are the solution to the epidemic of chronic disease.

Chapter 8
Reference List

About NIH: NIH Budget. National Institutes of Health (NIH). National Institutes of Health (NIH), 2005

Phase 3 Clinical Trial Costs Exceed $26,000 per Patient. Life Sciences World, 2006.

Amgen Pharmaceutical Manufacturing Facility, United States of America. Net Resources International, 2011.

Clinical Operations: Accelerating Trials, Allocating Resources and Measuring Performance. Business Intelligence Firm Cutting Edge Information, 2011.

National Diabetes Statistics, 2011: New Cases of Diagnosed Diabetes. National Diabetes Information Clearinghouse. National Diabetes Information Clearinghouse, 2011.

Peanuts and Peanut Butter Fun-Facts. National Peanut Board. National Peanut Board, 2011.

Barlett, DL, et al. "Why Drugs Cost So Much / The Issues '04: Why We Pay So Much for Drugs." Time Magazine U.S. 4 Feb. 2004.

Dairman, T. Exubera Inhaled Insulin Discontinued. R.A. Rapaport Publishing, Inc., 2010.

Fugh-Berman, A. and S. Batt. "This may sting a bit": cutting CME's ties to pharma. Pharmaceutical Industry Disclosure Practices, 2006.

Haddad, J. The Pharmaceutical Industry's Influence on Physician Behavior and Health Care Costs. San Francisco Medical Society, 2011.

Masia, N. The Cost of Developing a New Drug: New wonder medicines come from years of research, high costs. U.S. Department of State's Bureau of International Information Programs, 2011.

Newman, R. "Why Health Insurers Make Lousy Villains." Us News & Money 2008.

The Congress of the United States, Congressional Budget Office. Research and Development in the Pharmaceutical Industry. The Congress of the United States, Congressional Budget Office, 2010.

$$\Sigma$$

CHAPTER 9

Physicians: Following the Money Trail

Tommy and Yuki dreamed about becoming doctors. They told their dreams to their mom, their dad, their brothers and sisters, their schoolmates, and their teachers. In fact, they told everyone they knew what they wanted to be when they grew up. They wanted to help others, and make a lot of money. Tommy's and Yuki's dreams are part of the American experience and culture. They relate directly to the idea that incentives drive our behavior. These incentives start very young. Something in our lives motivates us to modify our behavior for the accomplishment of a long-term goal. This can be seen clearly in the course children take on their way to becoming Dr. Do-good's.

For the sake of discussion, assume that both Tom and Yuki decide they want to become physicians during their freshmen year in high school. To achieve their dream, they will need to finish high school (4 years), complete their undergraduate degree (4 years) attend medical school (4 years) and complete at least one or two years in an internship (2 years). 14 years after beginning high school, they will be able to hang out their shingles as physicians and begin to practice medicine on their own.

Money is a huge factor in this dream. The average debt for a medical school graduate can exceed $150,000. Depending on how long it takes to pay down the loan, the total amount may exceed $300,000. This amounts to a monthly payment of two to three thousand dollars. During their training some doctors work as many as 80 hours a week and receive an amount slightly above the family poverty level—around $35,000 to $45,000 a year—for salary. This calculates to around $11.00 an hour. This picture would frighten most of us if we knew we had to experience the pressure of performing as a physician in training and, at the same time, handle a huge debt load. What then drives Tom and Yuki to put in the long years of study and to take on the huge burden of debt?

Money is one answer. Money does make this world go around. Money is the incentive. Compared to other countries in the world, the average US physician makes $50,000 a year more. In the U.S., a new general practitioner, on average, makes over $150,000 dollars a year. The average specialist can make over $200,000 dollars a year. A starting cardiologist can make over $250,000; a new neurosurgeon, $350,000. Money is the answer, money is the incentive, and money allows the system to work. Taking these incentives into consideration, it becomes apparent that although we may dream of becoming doctors just like Tom and Yuki, money becomes a key motivation to succeed.

Staying motivated requires more than just having a distant reward. It requires reinforcement, consistency and predictability. Long term motivation is maintained by goal achievement and strong mentoring. It is achieved when the path is clear, rewards are frequent, and the prize is certain. This is why incentives work so well with motivating many children to become doctors. There is additional motivation for Tom and Yuki. Roughly 50% of students who apply to medical school will not be accepted. Hyper-competitive medical school entrance processes produce a fear-of-loss motivation for those stretching for doctor-hood. Each day of the 14 years of schooling, Yuki and Tom are immersed in a demanding environment, and are reminded of the need to do well (or else). Their motivation is constant, reinforced (sometimes by fear), and is predictable. Based on exam scores and grades, they receive regular reminders of how they are progressing.

Interestingly, compare Tommy's and Yuki's incentives to become doctors to the culture of motivation that prevents us from losing our beta cells from overeating and inactivity. The situations are polar opposites. There are no hope-to-gain monetary rewards to keep us healthy. We will not be paid $200,000 a year to remain in good shape for 14 years. As freshmen in high school, if we told our dream to be healthy to our friends, our family, our school mates, and our teachers, we would get a strange look, or at best, a pat on the head. There are no reinforcements to achieve this goal, no regular exams, and no grades to make us proud. Our path to health is strewn with delightful calorie temptations and television. At our graduation, there is no one cheering us on because we are in our ideal weight category.

As a result, we fall flat; actually, we fall fat. Our environment conspires against us. We have fatty meals at home, especially if we live in certain ethnic homes. We eat in fat-drenched restaurants, hang around with fatty friends, and pack around junk food to be cool. Contrasting the incentive structures for realizing our dream of becoming a doctor versus the dream of becoming a health conscious adult redirects us back to the financial incentives concept.

The opening example in this chapter places us in a position to carefully examine how we can change our incentive structure with the support of the types of motivations that produce our outstanding physicians. In this chapter, you will also learn about the monetary incentives embedded in our physician medical industry, and how these incentives determine how and where our care is delivered. This is critically important, because physician costs make up 20% of the total cost of healthcare in the United States. Understanding these incentives provides a necessary insight into creating and maintaining a world-class physician industry. This industry needs to support our efforts to stay healthy. Our physicians' recommendations are paramount to our following a healthy lifestyle.

Unfortunately, because of the nature of monetary incentives, many of us do not have affordable access to physician care. In fact, where individuals are the sickest, we have the fewest physicians. We discussed this earlier in relation to endocrinology specialists. We can understand why this may be the case: incentives. Physicians must earn a high salary to pay for their educational expenses and debt load. Can poor folks help them accomplish this faster than the rich folks? It does not take an economist to answer this question.

Physicians generally migrate to where they can earn the most money. They do this not just geographically; they accomplish this by migrating into specialty medicine. As noted earlier, some specialists make twice the income of general practitioners. There is strong competition among residents for positions in specialty programs, and much weaker competition for those in general or family medicine. Specialists tend to establish practices in high-income areas, where there is a strong private and cash-paying reimbursement base. Most specialists avoid high Medicaid areas, where reimbursement is the lowest and private insurance rates are suppressed by managed care health plans.

Physician monetary incentives compound the health challenges of our ethnic and poorer populations. Not only do our ethnic-community food cultures and activity-level cultures impact our health, but our lack of physician access does as well. Across almost all medical care parameters, poorer communities do less well in terms of fighting chronic diseases like diabetes, kidney disease, asthma, and heart disease. These facts are well-researched and available in multiple sources, both government and private.

Here is how to fix physician access problems

Something you may not know is that Medicare pays for the salaries of all medical students as they go through their residency (although this is not a high salary, as discussed above). Tax dollars also go to support in-state medical schools. Federal tax dollars go to research grants that provide substantial funding for teaching hospitals. Tax dollars support Medicare and Medicaid. Surprisingly, we also find that all of these huge student loans that cover the costs of medical school (and most other school loans) are obtained by going through the U.S. federal government loan program, a part of the U.S. Department of Education.

This is all good medicine and good government, but it also means that our tax dollars go to underwrite a physician's education <u>and income</u>. In essence, our tax dollars are backing the risk of loaning money to medical students, so they can become physicians. Tax dollars also pay to conduct the research that physicians do at universities where medical students are trained. Tax dollars are used to reimburse physicians for the care they give our seniors. We, the tax payers of the United States, provide the bulk of the monetary incentives that motivate physicians to acquire the education that propels them to become members of one of the highest-paid professions in the country (if not the world). And yet, where are they when we need them? They (generally speaking) are serving the richer and healthier part of our population.

As in the military, when someone is supported in their medical degree, they need to pay back with time in service. The incentive goes like this: we pay for you; you pay us back in your time where we need you to serve. Serve where you are needed, or where you are ordered to go by your commanding officer. There is no commanding officer in front of a fully-trained physician to direct them where to practice. There is only the commanding monetary opportunity.

Therefore, the time has come to consider a formal community service role for physicians. Physicians, who by their very training used the resources of the country's tax payers to become educated, need to donate more of their time and their talents to serve the poor. Not at their own discretion, but at the discretion of the government. This is the same government that guarantees their education loan and guarantees their reimbursement when treating the elderly Medicare patient as well as the poor Medicaid patient.

For physicians, what does this community service role look like? Simply put, in this community service model, approximately five percent of a physician's time and practice should be reserved to treat the underserved. One day in 18, (roughly three to four weeks a year), physicians should work at a county clinic in an area designated by the state health department. Physicians would be required to reserve a minimum of five percent of their practice for Medicaid patients, five percent for Medicare, and a final five percent for the uninsured. Substantial fines would be charged for physicians who do not comply. The fines are necessary motivators for physician compliance.

This proposed solution effectively can be built from the approximate universe of 700,000 physicians in the U.S. These physicians could be deployed at the discretion of the State Department of Health. They can cover underserved areas of the community, especially those that are being most affected by the epidemic of diabetes or other costly chronic diseases. This amount of donated time is roughly equal to

35,000 physician-equivalents. In other words, this proposed incentive system would generate 700 physician-equivalents per state. Currently there is a shortage of 14,000 physicians in the U.S., or 280 physicians per state, with a projected shortfall of over 1000 physician equivalents per state by 2015. This shortage represents millions of patients that are without adequate physician access.

We need to ensure that we have enough physicians to be available to meet the demands of covering our at risk populations. Part of the incentive package to create the physician community service core, could be the lowering of the loan repayment interest rate and delaying the loan repayment schedule. Reducing the interest rate and rescheduling a payment plan may equal tens of thousands of dollars reduction in the repayment of the loan. This action takes a substantial load off the graduating medical student and provides an avenue for them to perform community service. This loan re-structuring could be part of the incentive package that requires physicians to participate in supporting the underserved part of the population.

Logistically, the community service program seems impossible to implement, based on where physicians currently reside. We cannot expect them to drive hundreds of miles to treat patients every month. Realistically, we may need additional technology to support this incentive. Fortunately, most, if not all, of the required technology is available. Physicians, with the help of a technician, can remotely conduct a patient exam as if they themselves were in the room. A full-color video camera, with audio, and with all of the patient's vitals reported in real time, is transmitted over the internet. The transmission is within a top secret protocol, fully private and completely secure. This technology is currently on the market. It enables physicians to remotely examine a patient, formulate a diagnosis, and create a treatment plan, all from a clinic near to their regular practice location. In principle, this technology maximizes the physician's time, and allows for our incentive community service project to become a reality.

Out of Balance Physician Incentives (Kwok et al., 2011)

Growing research now attests to the fact that physicians may possibly order unnecessary procedures and tests, especially for those at the close of life. *The Lancet* reports that, "The rate at which they [Medicare patients at the end of life] undergo surgery varies substantially with age and region and might suggest discretion in healthcare providers' decisions to intervene surgically at the end of life." Furthermore, the variation in the frequency of surgery was correlated to the number of hospital beds, and the amount of Medicare spending.

This report indicates that physicians may be overly optimistic in suggesting that surgeries will be successful in either prolonging life, or improving the quality of life of senior patients, especially those who do not have that much more time to live. According to *The Lancet* researchers, approximately:

- 30 percent of senior patients underwent a surgical procedure in the last year of life.
- 20 percent of senior patients underwent a surgical procedure in the last month of life.

- 10 percent of senior patients went through a surgical procedure in the last week of life.

Examining physician incentives provides a clue to this remarkable finding. By the very nature of their specialty, surgeons are reimbursed by their invoiced procedures. In order to make money (and pay back their loans), a surgeon needs to operate. The more they operate, the more money they make and the faster their loans are repaid.

From an incentive standpoint, consider that Medicare does not allocate resources based on life-ending probabilities (thank goodness). Also, Medicare does not play the role of God. It seems that the analysis on whether a particular surgery will extend a life of a senior patient is left up to the family and to the doctor with whom they entrust the life of their loved one. This common situation demonstrates that surgeons, along with a high percentage of Medicare patients, routinely face a perverse incentive, as described by the result of the above research. Surgeons are faced with the dilemma to operate, even when there is a significant chance the patient will die within the first month following the operation. This is a moral hazard inherent in our current Medicare reimbursement structure.

To further support this claim of perverse incentives and moral hazards, evidence shows that poor patients, those that cannot pay, tend not to have the surgeries they need. Although it may seem a moral and noble idea to try to prolong life at any cost, perverse incentives may need to be removed or modified. As it stands now, the process is prejudicial in nature, favoring the surgeons and the wealthiest seniors, while disadvantaging the poor. The decision-making process is left in the hands of the surgeons, who give their professional opinions to the family. The family most likely will follow the surgeons' advice—from whom else can they find an answer to whether their loved one has a chance to live longer? Perhaps we may all need to pray more to solve this question.

The point of this discussion is not to reform this decision-making process, but to inform the reader that resources are grossly misallocated using the current form of incentives, in which surgeons make most of the decisions. Preventing one half of the *unnecessary* end-of-life Medicare surgeries frees hundreds of millions of dollars to address preventable chronic diseases with new incentives that may stop epidemics like diabetes. Reducing the unnecessary procedures may allow for these dollars to be re-allocated within Medicare. With these funds, Medicare could, in turn, chose to assist in educating more general practice physicians and the specialists that are critical to treating diabetes. In the future, with proper incentives, patients needing end-of-life surgeries may avoid the need for surgery in the first place if they have adequate access to preventive care directed through primary care physicians.

Fixing this perverse, misaligned incentive for *unnecessary* surgery procedures is simple: cut the reimbursement rate for surgeons and for hospitals whose senior patients die within one month of a procedure. To be fair, this cut could be tiered based on the age of the patient and the underlying diseases. Both of these factors directly predict mortality. Medicare is in possession of the end-of-life statistics that can be studied and analyzed to create such a protocol. Creating this simple scale, based on national statistics, may eliminate the majority of the perverse incentives. The physician and hospital incentive aligns with true medical need and medical quality. Family members and patients can review the statistics themselves and make a more informed decision on how to best help their senior loved one.

In a broader sense, behavioral economics predicts this surgical procedure outcome. The surgeon has a clear path to a reward. The path is reinforced daily, not just from a monetary point of view, but from an intrinsic point of view. The surgeon is thanked by the family for doing all that is humanly possible to extend life. And, in some cases, lives are extended due to the intervention. A surgeon is then rewarded handsomely for their expertise. Given these circumstances, the outcomes showing unnecessary procedures are predictable.

As reported in an earlier chapter, prolonging life with unnecessary procedures that cause pain and suffering, need not be rewarded. Those that die within a month of having surgery generally may not experience greater quality of life, nor may they enjoy the benefits of family and loved ones being near them. They are stuck in the hospital with a surgical wound. At thirty days, most, as seniors, would be struggling through the recovery process. They may even die in the hospital, not in the comfort of their own home. For many of us, making it out of this life gracefully will not be possible due to the perverse incentives creating unrealistically portrayed positive outcomes for end-of-life surgical procedures.

Physicians may need to be reimbursed based on adherence to guidelines. Rates of unnecessary procedures in senior populations would dramatically drop if economic incentives were in place to encourage surgeons to help families so their loved ones peacefully die at home. Instead of paying a surgeon simply for cutting, we need to modify incentives and pay them additionally for the positive outcome of a patient dying comfortably at home. Removing the silo incentive of surgery and adding a new one of equal financial benefit to the physician will quickly change this paradigm. This change is the right thing to do for patients and will dramatically reduce costs and improve quality. Economic principles prove their might yet again.

In the case of possible unnecessary surgery, we have proved a point and offered a solution. This type of procedure basis for physician income is not simply a case for surgeons to consider. It is rampant throughout government-reimbursed healthcare. All specialists earn the majority of their income from procedures. If the correct incentives are deduced, created, and benchmarked from the medical literature, we can multiply the savings throughout the Medicare system. The federal government has embarked on a bold new approach to healthcare financing, one that has its underpinnings in comparative effectiveness research (CER). This approach offers a potential tipping point, a real breakthrough for incentive science.

Comparative Effectiveness Research (CER)

The government considers comparative effectiveness research as:

> ...evidence that compares the benefits and harms of alternative methods [procedures] to prevent, diagnose, treat, and monitor a clinical condition or to improve the delivery of care. The purpose of CER

is to assist consumers, clinicians, purchasers, and policy makers to make informed decisions that will improve health care at both the individual and population levels; (Committee on Comparative Effectiveness Research Prioritization & Institute of Medicine, 2009)

In laymen terms, CER means that the government will hire researchers to compare the effectiveness and safety of competing procedures to determine the one that produces the best outcome. The most successful procedures will merit the crowning endorsement of the government. The government is looking for the best outcome, not the cheapest alternative. This is a major step forward in science, and represents the beginning of the systematic benchmarking of best practices across all procedures in medicine. The faster this is accomplished, the sooner proper incentives can be established in the marketplace for physicians to follow.

Currently, the setting of reimbursement rates for certain procedures is arcane and rife with misguided incentives. This is another situation where economic processes may be misaligned because they possibly change the treatment course of patients with chronic diseases like diabetes. The process may divert limited resources for disease prevention to physician specialty income. The area we are referring to is the process used in the setting of Medicare rates for procedures. The system for setting rates for procedures is managed in part by the American Medical Association (AMA), its members, and its member organizations. In this semi-public and well-documented procedural process, approximately 30 physicians and advisors help <u>set the rates</u> for Medicare medical procedure reimbursement.

There is a challenge made in the literature to the AMA's involvement. Recent gains in funding procedures for specialists may have resulted in funding reductions for preventive care and general practitioners. This reimbursement imbalance is evidenced by the amount specialists are paid versus the amount a family practitioner is paid: nearly a 30% differential. Examining recent increases in physician reimbursement rates for certain procedures in certain areas of the country may point to excesses.

The AMA asserts that the process is fair and open, although the rate-setting meeting itself is conducted behind closed doors. This policy is to protect the privacy of the volunteer participants. The output of the meeting and the notes are made public. The reality is: the government accepts the vast majority of this AMA committee's recommendations. It follows their advice as applied to constructing physician reimbursement rates for procedures billed by physicians. It may be difficult for the government to aggressively question the committee recommendations after the government encourages them, in the first place, to come up with the needed recommendations. Revealed herein is yet another perverse economic incentive.

Rate-setting needs to be the purview of evidence-based medicine. Rate-setting needs to be independent of the perverse incentives that occur when those that set the rates are those same doctors that bill for the procedure itself. Economic principles, including measurements of the quality of life, need to reveal the most efficient procedure in the market. Economics uncover the most effective procedures and these need to be selected by market forces that offer fair supply and demand scenarios. Realistically, some procedures are monopolistic and may use patented technology, etc. Yet the procedures need to be compared to the next-best alternative.

The entire schema of procedure reimbursement for specialists may need to be examined against a greater investment in understanding preventive-care science, including finding effective patient incentives. These incentives may prevent the need for the majority of procedures in the first instance. As discussed earlier, 80 percent of diabetes is preventable.

US Physicians: the best in the world (?)

Arguably, U.S. physicians are the best in the world. By any standard, medical degrees from the U.S. are recognized worldwide as an excellent credential. By default, this degree grants a U.S. trained and licensed physician privileges to practice medicine in many parts of the world (assuming no language barriers). Why? Because the U.S. is recognized as the source for the majority of new science regarding most disease states, and is the originator of most new technologies and procedures. Simply put, the U.S. establishes the best standard of care practices. As a result, if you are trained to these standards, your credentials are held in high esteem the world over.

We might be tempted to think that if we have the best trained doctors, we should have the best medical outcomes. This logic, however, is flawed, and points to the issue of physician and patient incentives. A report on healthcare quality, comparing the U.S. results to other developed countries, found the following:

> Instead the picture emerges from the information available on technical quality and related aspects of health system performance is a mixed bag, with the United States doing relatively well in some areas... and less well in others – such as mortality from conditions amenable to prevention and treatment. Many Americans would be surprise by the findings from studies showing that U.S. health care is not clearly superior to that received by Canadians... it is often held that the U.S. strength lies in state-of-art, technically oriented care, especially focused on "rescue" care, rather than care for more routine acute and chronic conditions [such as diabetes]. (Docteur & Berenson, 2009)

The findings of the report confirm our discussion that while U.S. physicians lead the world in interventional procedures using cutting edge technologies, they do not outshine their worldwide peers in the rate of successful treatment of chronic diseases. This may be partially explained through behavioral economics. U.S. physicians are highly compensated and motivated by the billing of medical procedures. The newer the procedure, the more costly and greater the invoice is for reimbursement. This incentive structure increases the demand for new technology development and creates a market force for the utilization of novel technology. U.S. doctors make more money on diagnosis and interventions <u>than they make on preventing and treating chronic conditions like diabetes.</u>

This report does not conclude that the U.S. physicians deliver substandard care. It simply points out the strengths and weaknesses of our system of incentives.

Ironically, there is a simple economic fix to these market forces that undervalue prevention and treatment and overvalue procedures and technology development. The economic solution is placed squarely on the patient, not the physician. We need to increase the incentives for patients to be compliant with their doctors' prescribed treatment plans, so that they avoid the need for more expensive procedures. Americans can have a high sense of confidence that their physician is prescribing appropriate care when it comes to a chronic disease like diabetes. After all, the treatment guidelines are world-class. Although we are confident regarding the information we are provided by our doctors, at the same time we also remain generally non-compliant to prescribed treatment plans.

All of the prior chapters in this book point to the reasons why we are failing in the area of compliance to doctor orders for the care of our beta cells and diabetes. This section of the book describes in more detail how physicians can assist us to become compliant. This chapter's information does not suggest that we need more self-control, more disease education, more diagnostic procedures, or more diet and exercise training by our doctors. Doctors and their staff are simply not resourced to provide the amount of hand-holding required for us to work through the roadblocks in our lives that prevent our compliance.

Rather, this chapter is dedicated to describing the incentive interface between our insurance companies, our employers, and our providers. It is an interchange that motivates us to closely follow our own treatment plan. The plan that is right for us. To be effective, the plan's incentives need to be clear, frequently reinforced, goal oriented, and mentored. To illuminate this process, an example patient's journey is important to consider.

Manuel

Manuel, a 45-year-old construction worker, complained to his doctor about his symptoms. By conducting routine blood tests, the doctor promptly diagnosed him as a patient with diabetes. The tests were inexpensive and ensured a definitive diagnosis. The doctor's staff informed Manuel that his company offered insurance incentives that could assist Manuel with his illness. The doctor understood this information because Manuel's insurance paid the doctor handsomely for closely following Manuel, especially if he could help him avoid going to the hospital or needing expensive imaging as a result of diabetes complications. The reimbursement was significant and covered the time his staff needed to spend with Manuel to educate him on important issues.

The discussion Manuel had with the doctor's staff was not just about diet and exercise, but also included special attention discussing his copayments for hospitalization, procedures, doctor visits, as well as for his medicines. Costs for all could drastically increase (by 30%), if the doctor's orders were not closely followed. The staff also asked Manuel if he had a phone that can receive a text message, which he confirmed.

In fact, if he did not own a phone, his insurance company would provide a phone. Manuel was informed that his insurance company provided free disease-management and wellness programs. Manuel liked the idea that these messages and instructions would be delivered via his phone, or via his personal computer. In some cases, a health educator would be in touch. Manuel would regularly receive important and reinforcing messages and education.

This wellness and disease management program enabled success with his doctor's prescribed treatment plan. At the same time, the insurance company was fully informed of his progress. Tracking his progress and informing his physician allowed Manuel to stay healthier and avoid costly procedures and hospital stays. All of this is information was kept strictly confidential. Manuel's employer was not informed, unless Manuel chose to do so.

The employer pre-arranged for Manuel and the entire workforce to receive the best care and to be offered the strongest incentives possible to be compliant. They knew from the data that this approach was the most cost-effective approach for their employee population because, in part, it increased productivity and morale. The employer had negotiated these incentives prior to the onset of Manuel's illness, with the expert assistance of the insurance company. The insurance company proceeded to negotiate the incentives with their nationally contracted physician network. Again, all of the information Manuel shared regarding his care and his compliance with the doctor's treatment plan was kept confidential by the insurance company and by his provider.

The insurance company successfully negotiated a rich reimbursement for the primary care physicians. The physicians were pleased to agree, under these new terms and conditions, to also facilitate the reporting of patient compliance. They reported vitals (including weight loss/gain), appointment attendance, educational class attendance, lab values, and prescription refills. This complete picture of patient compliance, gathered by insurance companies and physicians, demonstrated how Manuel and other patients just like him responded to incentives that were proven to reduce care costs and improve care quality. Please recall that if Manuel purposefully, voluntarily, and willfully did not follow the treatment plan, he was at risk for paying additional premiums.

The end of the story is positive. Manuel continued to control his diabetes. Compared to other patients with diabetes from other companies, he missed fewer days of work due to his illness and he used less medical resources, including fewer procedures and less hospital care. He used more medicine on average because he is more compliant. He took his medicine as directed and refilled the prescription on time. This prescription-cost increase to the system is far outweighed by his continued avoidance of costly surgeries, dialysis, and hospitalizations. Everyone was pleasantly surprised by these results except the economist, who totally expected these cost savings from the beginning.

Economic principles are constantly tweaked over the backs of physicians and their practices. Some notable examples from the recent past include managed care, pay for performance, quality incentives, specialized risk contracts, fee for service, drug audits, and hospital costs sharing... on, and on it goes. And still, the epidemic of diabetes grows.... Costs for the disease are accelerating. You may be bored to tears reviewing each of these strategies in depth, only to find, in the end, that the missing ingredient to control costs in all of the strategies <u>is the patient's financial responsibility</u>.

None of these strategies and experiments in physician-remuneration assisted patients with the motivation they needed to be more compliant. These experiments did not incentivize the patient to reduce costs. None of these economic strategies, as administered through physician networks, simultaneously addressed the issue of non-compliant patients. There have been, to date, no available mechanisms for insurance companies to engage the patient and the doctor in a manner that incentivizes the patient. This engagement needs to include monitoring, incenting, and shaping compliance behavior to ensure adherence to the doctor's prescribed treatment protocols. The patient incentives must be closely monitored by the physicians in order to assure the best-quality outcomes. Physicians by themselves would find it impossible to establish proper patient financial incentives, due to the fact that they do not control the benefit design that supports patient compliance. Consider this list of agencies physicians must comply with if they happen to venture into patient-compliance incentives.

Patient incentives must be congruent with the policies of Health and Human Services, Centers for Disease Control and Prevention, the Federal Drug Administration, Veterans

Administration, Medicare, Medicaid, State Insurance Commissioners, American Medical Association, hospital associations, pharmacy associations, nursing associations, union leadership, quality organizations, State Health Departments, County Health Departments, corporate ethics committees, privacy advocacy organizations, and patient advocacy groups. Recognize that in the end, the incentive needs to be signed off by the patients themselves, and in some cases, the patients' families. Neither physicians nor any other singular entity can negotiate all of this bureaucracy, though it needs to happen if we are to stop diabetes.

These organizations provide outstanding service, education, and support. They are the backbone of quality in our medical industry and community. They protect patients. They advocate for patients. They care for patients. However, one thing they have never done well is stopping the diabetes epidemic by properly incentivizing patient behavior as measured by patient compliance. These organizations do not have the science, the skill sets, or the legal mandate to accomplish this feat. Nor can they alone overcome our food culture. No one has the legal mandate. It falls into a no-fly zone, into uncharted waters. Exploring this "zone" deeply and broadly can lead us to a place where we can find and implement solutions big enough to take down diabetes. Physicians, as the true advocates of patient care, need to lead the discussion.

The major purpose of this chapter is to provide evidence that physicians are a singularly powerful source available for us to begin to solve the economic problems inherent with the spread of diabetes. Before we can fully engage this expert community, we must ensure that their incentives are aligned with the right solutions. There is evidence that physician incentives, as they stand today, may direct scarce resources away from dealing with the root causes of the epidemic. The evidence points to the fact that too many unnecessary procedures are performed in our Medicare population, while inadequate incentives are provided for primary care physicians and endocrinologists. Primary care incentives need to align with personal incentives for patients. The solution to this mix of issues is aligning the expertise of public and private insurance with public and private employers in order to provide benefit designs powerful enough to motivate and support patient compliance.

This is no simple task. This process cannot take more money out of an already financially strapped health care system. It takes a coordinated plan. It requires a plan that breaks down the barriers to patient involvement and patient responsibility in their own care. A strategy and plan is needed that determines success more in terms of prevention and less in terms of rescuing non-compliant patients. This is a plan and strategy that simply re-aligns incentives in order for patients to be supported. To date, the patient, in spite of all of our best intentions and the efforts of the best-trained medical professionals in the world, has been left out of the financial incentive motivation. There is an easy way through this, however. It is to follow the money trail. Those who hold the purse strings to treating our preventable chronic illnesses can step up and create benefit designs that strongly encourage full patient engagement. They can modify physician compensation away from unnecessary procedures to overseeing patient incentives. Public payers may need to follow private payers in establishing best practices for patient incentives programs.

Patients learning about their responsibilities are part of best practices. Patients discussing the plan with their physicians are part of best practices. The grand key is physician reimbursement for effective oversight of their patient's compliance to their prescribed treatment plan. Patients need to be held financially responsible to the payer and to the provider. Best practices will minimize hospitalizations and unnecessary procedures. Once best practices are in place and the incentives are immediate, consistent, and rewarding, we will begin to stop diabetes in its tracks.

- So predicts the science of behavioral economics.

Chapter 9
Reference List

Committee on Comparative Effectiveness Research Prioritization & Institute of Medicine (2009). *Initial National Priorities for Comparative Effectiveness Research*. The National Academies Press.

Docteur, E. and Berenson, RA (2009). How Does the Quality of U.S. Health Care Compare Internationally? Timely Analysis of Immediate Health Policy Issues. Urban Institiute.
www.urban.org/uploadedpdf/411947_ushealthcare_quality.pdf

Kwok, A., Semel, M., Lipsitz, S., Bader, A., Barnato, A., & Gawande, A. A. (10-15-2011). "The intensity and variation of surgical care at the end of life: a retrospective cohort study." The Lancet 378[9800], 1408-1413. 11-28-2011.

$$\Sigma$$

CHAPTER 10

Healthcare Incentives: Putting the Puzzle Together

<u>My Parents are Slender Geniuses</u>

As a child, I loved to go to the circus. I loved the traveling carnivals, the ones where you had to buy tickets for each ride. I never had enough money in my pocket to go on any of the exceptionally fun rides. So, what did I do – I begged my parents for more money. Their help was not forth coming. They said if I wanted to ride the merry-go-round, I would have to earn the money for it on my own – no micro loans either! The fact is I never did earn that extra money. I never put my plan together to mow the grass, paint the fence, or least of all, vacuum the family room, just so I could ride the "wild thing", the next time the circus came to town. Only, my empty pockets reminded me to earn money for the circus.

Alas, America has opened the gate to a real food carnival culture, one that is inexpensive for all to enjoy. Historically, food purchases made up 30 percent of a household budget. Currently, food purchases account for only 6 or 7 percent of our household budget. We can buy all of the cotton candy we want, and still have some left over for the big ride. What is stopping us now – nothing, certainly not boomer baby parents.

The time has come for us to recognize that our wealth is killing us prematurely. Our freedom to buy inexpensive, high fat, high sugar and high salt food – our metabolism merry-go round - is choking our arteries, killing our pancreases, and stimulating cancer cells. Our wealth may bankrupt us, our families, and our health system. How ironic – our wealth may cause us to go bankrupt. The food circus is in full gear and there is no parent at the ticket gate.

When I was lucky enough to go out for a meal, my parents would pay for everything except sugared drinks or desserts. They explained I could buy unhealthy food for myself, with my own money (which I seldom had in my pocket). Their job was to buy their children healthy food. If I could find a way to pay for my own treats, dessert or candy, etc., that was fine by them – only, I had to pay the consequences. My parents were slender geniuses. They knew that if having the things that were inherently bad for my body was truly important to me, I would need to purchase them with my own funds. Needless to say, I had few cavities as a kid.

What happened when I became an adult? From the time I graduated high school, until I hit forty years old, I gained 45 pounds (similar to national statistics). Some of those pounds are with me today – despite a decade of losing and gaining weight. The simple fact is – my parents were no longer the gatekeepers of healthy eating incentives and healthy choices. With the rest of America, my food costs, as a percentage of my annual salary, dropped to below 10%. I could reasonable buy and eat anything I liked, and wanted. Not only that, since I was traveling 30% of the time, my employer paid for my food. I got fat, along with America. I surmise that you are not much different.

This text introduces economically sound, inexpensive strategies to address the cultural problem of relatively cheap fatty food. These strategies, if applied across our culture, can act as the surrogate gatekeeper of our health. The strategy does not cost any more money. Like all good things, the strategy is simple: assist us in making better choices by applying stronger economic incentives. The new parent that will save our heartland and our economy is the parent of health incentives.

Perhaps, it is time to create healthy gate keepers and processes across our culture, in our homes and schools, with our employers, and imbed them in our health insurance benefits. Health incentives outlined throughout *Dianomics* can solve the problem of diabetes and the premature loss of our beta cells. These incentives are the economic, dietary and behavioral tactics, targeting the sources of excess fat, sugar, and salt in our diet. These motivators have the capacity to shrink our health costs, and positively impact our resiliency by preventing heart disease, strokes, and diabetes.

Dianomics changes the discussion of our collective health by presenting ideas regarding how the health industry can engage with corrective action with individuals, families, communities, governments, pharmaceutical companies, insurance companies, employers, and physicians supporting one another. The nucleus of this discussion is the idea of financial incentives powerfully aligned to help us modify our consumption patterns. These are incentives that will eventually enable us to lose unwanted fat and reduce our healthcare costs. Employers, insurance companies, physicians, and communities will benefit from this approach.

What has been tried in the way of incenting patients, and what are the results to date of that effort? Five years ago, an exhaustive worldwide literature search on this subject was conducted in England(Dixon, 2008). The study found the following:

> In summary, based on the body of theoretical work there is reason to believe that motivation and confidence are key determinants of behavior change. *However, there are few known effective interventions for each of the behaviors examined here – smoking, exercise and diet. Most of the interventions that are implemented are not explicit about how they work nor do they assess or report measures of motivation of self-efficacy.* Finally, there are very few studies that attempt to answer the question of why interventions change behavior by measuring both behaviors and the mediating variables. So, it is impossible to conclude whether the theories are in fact right. *None of the reviews identified measured cost-effectiveness so, it is not possible to conclude whether any of these interventions are worth the NHS investing in. [emphasis added]*

From a recent article in the *New England Journal of Medicine*, Dr. Volpp and co-authors note: "...evidence that differential premiums change health-related behavior is scant. Indeed we are unaware of any health insurance data that have convincingly demonstrated such effects." (Volpp, 2011)

There is general scientific evidence regarding the psychological components that enable substantial and sustained changes to the behaviors affecting our health. The three key components are:

1) Intrinsic, or internal self-motivation
2) Extrinsic, or external rewards or punishments
3) Self-confidence, we think we can change.

Most of the healthcare literature addressing incentives aligns with studying strategies relating to identifying the state of change that we are in - our intrinsic motivational state - and providing education in the form of written/verbal counseling to boost our self-confidence. This process is designed to reinforce the emotional touch stone of intrinsic motivation.

Along with this information, we may leave the doctor's office with a lab result highlighting our plight, including a possible impending health disaster. Even if we are diagnosed with a serious problem, providing information alone, without behavioral tactics, seems to be weakly helpful. Providing training around actual behavioral coping strategies, combined with information, produces a stronger, but still relatively weak patient change result. Additionally, studies rarely report statistics on how the educational intervention or behavioral coping strategies impact total healthcare costs. We are left wondering, do these strategies hold the key to our long term fiscal health – probably not.

Extrinsic motivators are another incentive category studied somewhat in the healthcare literature. These motivators rely on a carrot and stick approach, and are studied to a lesser extent in the patient health literature. The behavioral changes that result from extrinsic beneficial, financial incentives, such as winning a weight loss contest, or earning a minimal gift, seem difficult to assess in terms of the provable psychological impact of the incentive. A review on the literature suggests that such incentives, when they are substantial, do have a stronger impact than information alone, yet the change in behavior is short lived, and usually dies off once the extrinsic incentive is earned. In other words, the patient response is, "What have you done for me lately?"

The extrinsic motivation studies to date have inadequately structured incentives that produce minimal long term behavior change. Once earned, these weak incentives may fail to engage a powerful and sustained emotional response. Without intrinsic and extrinsic reinforcement, most of us lose our momentum to change. The science of extrinsic motivation with powerful incentives, enough to prevent this loss of momentum is understudied in the literature. To date, extrinsic healthcare incentives demonstrating successful behavior changes over a substantial period of time are simply not well explored or understood. Perhaps, we can find more information or examples of these principles from a very unlikely, non-scientific source.

Consider the case of the many celebrities that endorse health related products. We could lose 50 pounds too, if we were paid hundreds of thousands of dollars, and then pose in all of our glory for the praise of an adoring public. Not to mention, we would jump at all of the talk show appearance opportunities designed to promote our new book. We would bet our bottom <u>and</u> our last dollar. Celebrity weight loss exposés are an extreme case of extrinsic motivation. Yet, during interviews these newly slender celebrities say something like, "I did not do it for the money, I did it so I could feel better about myself, and have more energy." This statement, including the comment on wanting to feel better about something, describes an example of intrinsic motivation.

Certainly, the intrinsic motivation statement is real to the celebrity – but where's the beef? What actually got the celebrities off the couch and into celebrity health rehab? Was it the desire to feel better (intrinsic motivation) that sustained them through the torturous months of working out and eating less, or was it the desire to hit the bank with a fat check (extrinsic motivation)? You and I do not need a psychologist or an economist to answer these questions. Consider other celebrities weight loss woes. Once their endorsement contract ended, they swiftly gained their weight back. Perhaps their intrinsic motivation was not strong enough, or they lost their extrinsic motivation all together. The real question for America is: what will it take for us to permanently change?

- Will it take a feeling inside that we may want to change?
- Will it take our own nagging desire to lose weight?
- Will it be winning the lottery?

- Will I lose something I already have if I do not make this change?
- How much money would it take? $1,000, $100,000, or more…?
- Will we be poked by an alert employer's insurance company that analyzed our health risk assessment and found a serious issue we need to address?

Heaven forbid if it is the government that demands us to change!

The Law of the Super Shopper

Together, we can build our success rate for changing, by utilizing all of the success factors identified in the literature, combining the best elements of extrinsic and intrinsic motivation. Consider the "The law of the Super Shopper". It goes something like this:

Our super shopper selves hit the store floor in bargain mode. We begin the day by thinking, "If I do not shop today, I may miss out on using my discount coupon and my preferred shopper status." As we land at our favorite store, we speedily fly through the aisles with the greatest of ease. Before long, we sniff out the new jeans and cannot wait to try them on. We buy the jeans because they are part of a super-sale-event -90%-off with our preferred customer coupon. We remember we saw the same jeans featured in happy advertisements, modeled by gorgeous people we can only dream to look like. We hope we can look and feel just like the model.

Once home it is a match, we have a new look, the jeans fit well (although, a little tighter than we might have otherwise predicted), and boom we feel great. We throw out our old tired, beat up jeans. We look just fine, and we feel fantastic. We greet the weekend in high fashion. As a result of our new look, wonderful things happen. We charge into the dating scene, meet our soul mate, and land our dream job.

Here, we have the play-by-play framework for motivational success. We experience a twinge of concern, that we may lose our preferred customer status, if we don't use our coupon. We are extrinsically motivated by a once in a lifetime sales event, that may pass us by if we do not jump on the bandwagon. We enjoy confidence – we have cash in our pocket and have just lost five pounds. We are ready for change. We gain information - the advertisements and our friends told us that they themselves had already bought a pair of these jeans, and promised us that we too will look great in them. We seem to have found our intrinsic motivation – shopping helps beat the blues, and we really think it is time for us to do something for ourselves. As a result of all of the intrinsic and extrinsic motivators coming together, we can take courage and change our behavior. We go out-on-the-town, for the first time in several months, igniting our spirits, and cementing our positive schema for shopping as a means of improving our lives. We become unstoppable.

This accentuated behavior model of a super shopper seeking to change their life is a key to the financial rescue of the United States healthcare system. All of the critical elements in making lasting change are present, including: a fear of losing some preferred status, a readiness to change, a strong financial incentive, a confidence that our efforts will have the desired outcome, reliable information, frequent reinforcing by friends and family, financial resources, and finally, continued future benefits. By proudly wearing the jeans, the super shopper positively reinforces the buying decision. The reinforcement for the buying decision continues to grow as the super shopper's success in life continues in a positive direction.

We can all relate to this example, well, at least up to the point of living happily ever after. To support our change efforts, we can live _healthily_ ever after by harnessing all of these motivators. We can hit a home run. This is how we load the bases.

First Base: Medicare

The first base runner for our novel intervention is grandma. This sounds counter intuitive to the analogy, but since we are hitting a home run, grandma can walk the bases. Medicare is the driving force behind the impending financial distress of our current retiree health benefit structure. Hospital costs, in particular, make up the most immediate threat to the program. Economic estimates forecast all of the Medicare hospital funds will be used up in fifteen years. _Dianomics_ explains that there is a cost effective strategy involving the Medicare member's intrinsic desire to die, pain free, at home, with the extrinsic motivation to prepare for that eventuality by filing an advanced directive.

This is how the system will work. Each state will have a centralized secure advance directive repository for Medicare patients. This site facilitates easy access to filing a preapproved, legally binding advance directive. This directive is filed and accessed by phone, email, fax, mail, etc., or by live operator (the exception). As part of the benefit package each year, during open enrollment, every senior over 65 may complete (or have a legal advocate complete) an advanced directive, and file it with their state repository.

This action allows the beneficiary to receive Medicare at current rates. Choosing not to file an advanced directive allows beneficiaries to enroll in Medicare at a premium rate, albeit with substantially higher hospital stay co-payments, and deductibles. In addition, as part of the advance directive filing, all Medicare patients will be able to check a box which pre-approves them for end of life hospice program, when prescribed by a physician.

Physicians and their staff are critical to the implementation of healthcare incentives. Physician office staff members are a catalyst to this part of the *Dianomics* incentives program. They can be considered first base coaches. Physicians receive additional compensation for assisting seniors with filing advance directives in conjunction with their office visit. The office staff can complete the process, as a designated patient advocate. Advanced directive training is augmented with additional training on the advantages of hospice care, and how and when to prescribe this Medicare benefit. An accompanying incentive payment system will compensate physicians and their office staff for participating in this state-wide standardized process. Physicians will be compensated for proven effective prescribing, especially for Medicare patients.

Medicare patients (or their advocates) are informed of the advantages for remaining at home during the end of life period. An important advantage is reducing pain and suffering caused by unnecessary tests, procedures and operations. Surgeons, whose Medicare patients undergo an unnecessary surgical procedure in the last month of their life, may receive a greatly reduced fee for the surgery. Medicare can guide the surgeons in their decisions about whether or not to operate by creating this reimbursement policy. This reimbursement policy will prevent unnecessary surgeries, and can be reviewed in advance by utilizing up to date quality assurance data.

Medicare can utilize comparative effectiveness research data, including a standard measurement on quality of life, to assist families and their healthcare providers with timely decisions. The data is vetted and thoroughly reviewed by both informed patient advocates and expert panels, ensuring that proper incentives are in the system enabling reasonable end of life decisions by both the seniors and their families. With their doctor's advice, seniors make the best possible care decisions for themselves. Weeded out of Medicare are incentives that reward unnecessary procedures, especially those procedures that cause undue suffering, and do not extend the quality of life.

Second Base: Employers

A highly secure and effective second base winning strategy can be provided by our employers. Employers, covering insured workers and their dependents, are the heavy hitters of our health incentive. Employers engage all of us in the workplace on a daily basis. This is when and where our health is put to the test. Employers know when we call in sick, and when we are the most productive. They "get it" when we might need to be relieved as in the case of a beleaguered pitcher heading into the seventh inning. What we are talking about here does not mean our employer is going to trade us to another team, or fire us for an acute injury. This analogy is about employers engaging us early on, like at spring training, so we avoid a career altering, or a career ending injury to our beta cells.

Spring training at our employer's work place would look like something akin to reviewing last year's playbook. The employers have an effective tool - it is called the health risk assessment. This assessment provides us with a look at the results of our past dietary choices, as well as a look into the future risk of a chronic disease, like diabetes, or a terminal illness, such as lung cancer caused by smoking. This is where the employer calls in the hitting coach. The hitting coach, with the assistance of the state insurance commissioner, and the employer's selected insurance provider, can design a new and exciting health benefit. This new benefit includes intrinsic and extrinsic incentives created to help motivate us to change. This health benefit becomes our play action regimen. It has a name: Three Strikes and We are Out.

Here is how it works. If we, (and/or our dependent) are diagnosed with a preventable chronic disease like type 2 diabetes, we can enroll ourselves into an enhanced benefit design, all at no additional initial cost to us, or our family. We are provided with expert education for our condition. We are required to select a primary doctor to discuss a mutually agreed upon treatment plan for our chronic disease. The doctor is contracted with the insurance company to provide us with the nationally recognized best practice standard of care. If we follow this treatment plan, we will remain in the current benefit design. This plan is effective for the vast majority because it is simple, easily managed, and frequently rewarded. It even has a fear of loss element to its extrinsic motivation.

There are three ways, or three strikes, that cause a change to the incentivized insurance benefit plan. Each strike relates to motivating our full participation in our own treatment; the treatment we agree upon with our physician that would be best for our individual situation. Strike one occurs if we routinely fail to complete prescribed education classes, such as how to administer insulin, or how to stop smoking. Strike two occurs if we regularly miss laboratory appointments, or doctor appointments. These are appointments and laboratory analysis that are prescribed by our physician based on national standards and best practices. Strike three knocks us out of the current health benefit, and occurs if we do not stop smoking, or stop our excess weight gain. In other words, if we do not follow the doctor's orders, we strike out of our low cost benefit design. We automatically enroll into a substantially higher co-pay plan, one that directly reflects the costs of our purposeful non-adherence.

Aligning incentives to reward us at work for being healthy and productive is a critical key to the puzzle of incentives, and the reinforcement necessary to change our risky behaviors. Work is the place where our risky behavior is privately brought to our attention, not directly by our employer, but by our insurance provider. At work we may receive frequent reminders of how productive or unproductive we are compared to our peers. Sometimes these reminders are a direct result of preventable and costly chronic diseases. Work is a place where our hitting coach can straighten out our swing, and shape us into a power hitter. Employers can load second base.

Third Base: School

School is a place of beginnings, and should never be relegated to a third position. In this case, school is third place because it is closest to home base and the easiest base from which to score a run. Protecting our children from beta cell death is a ready-made score for us to work towards at school. Beta cell loss is an urgent issue, and it is at an epidemic level among children. Children are becoming children with diabetes at a faster rate than in any point in the history of the world. Schools are a rallying point, a tipping point. Schools are a zone where we can all safely stand together. We can all stand, with our children, on third base, and get them to home safely.

Schools are a place where parents and children have a voice. Perhaps, parents are the third base running coaches in our analogy. They can coach their child to run, when to run, how to run, how hard and how fast to run. They themselves can walk into the principal's office and ask – "How come my child is not running!" Parents can look around their neighborhood and say, "why are we feasting on fattening foods? Is this what we are serving at school?"

The parent, as a coach, would never allow their star athlete to train on the stuff of school vending machines, and some school lunch programs. Surely they would not let their child, their star athlete, spend days idling with little or no physical activity. These coaches, our parents, encourage the best out of their child, including an hour of physical activity every day. But, if all that is going on already, what could be missing from the training schedule? Yes, you got it, intrinsic and extrinsic incentives.

From the point of view of incentives, here is what third base, closest to home, looks like at school. Frequently reinforced, clearly understood, unencumbered, intrinsic and extrinsic rewarding incentives work the best for children. Rewarded healthy behavior can start at school. This can take the form of a gold star, peer recognition, team sports, physical activity completion, home room activities, healthy menu preparation, trophies and medals. A letter grade could be achieved on health subjects each week (frequent reinforcement). A child may come home and say, "Look Mom, this is what I achieved, an A in health this week, and, "Look friends, this is who I am - someone who likes the rewards associated with healthy choices."

Our children need to be protected at school from the epidemic of obesity and type 2 diabetes. Measurement of physical activity and weight is the gold standard of initial intervention. Weight is a surrogate marker for future disease, and beta cell death. The science around this fact is voluminous. Children at risk may need to see a professional health advocate, as if their life depended on it.

Guarded in this process, and made the highest priority, is the child's physiological health. In our baseball example this is similar to a third base coach protecting the runner's advancement. The runner cannot see all that is happening around them, they need to focus on getting safely home. Tailored behavior and environmental interventions, guided by professional services, are needed for children at risk.

Ensuring the right incentives are in place will prove to have the greatest impact. They will help our children run the fastest and score the most points. <u>Healthy behavior incentives are more important than health education to a child's future.</u>

Measuring and aggregating the location of at risk school children, facilitates targeted deployment of community and government resources and incentives. Powerful incentives engage schools and parents in prevention strategies that protect children from the subtlety dangerous trend of childhood obesity. Levied penalties may be appropriate for non-participation of schools and unresponsive parents. Positive incentives can take the form of required physical activity, mandatory parental education, lower tax subsides (both property and sales), and waived copayments at county health clinics. Withholding tax exemptions and matching state and federal tax dollars for non-compliant schools and parents are powerful extrinsic incentive penalties. Incentives need not cost more money. Incentives only need to be sufficient enough to ensure engagement, participation and results. A good third base coach can make this happen. They can shout, "Run Johnny, run!" and ensure that Johnny makes it safely home.

<u>Home Base: Where the game is eventually won or lost.</u>

Striding towards the batter's box and home base, we suddenly see our own child. Our child is the accumulation of our genes, our love, our coaching example, and their diet. Successfully swinging the bat and connecting with the ball depends greatly on what we have given them in life, and the impact of their home environment. We say a prayer when they are called on to hit a home run, because we know a part of their success is about what we have provided them as parents and role models. We cheer them on as they move confidently to the plate, dust off their cleats, and stare down the opposing team's pitcher.

This is where the rubber meets the road, and these are some of the hard questions that may ring in our ears. Do we recognize how and where health risks are lurking? What impact is my example of healthy eating and activity level providing my child; is it supportive, or less than supportive? What regular intrinsic incentives do we provide in our family that reinforce and reward good health (have we even ever stopped to consider this idea)? What extrinsic financial rewards do we have to help maintain our child's healthy choices and forward momentum? We know what is right, but do we reinforce our positive decisions with regular recognition during and right after our child makes good choices? Sometimes just knowing what is good for us, is not sufficient to protect our children. Understanding motivation may need to be thought of more as a requirement than an afterthought.

Will power is not always enough to keep us and our children on a spring training schedule, nor is basic education. Our environment is daily overwhelming our children with poor alternatives and choices. In order to maintain good health, my son or daughter may need a coaching environment filled with intrinsic and extrinsic motivations. Pinching our waist lines can help us recognize whether or not we are optimizing our coaching abilities and deploying incentives. Sixty percent of us could probably use a refresher parenting course on healthy eating and activity, and the incentives that help us make appropriate choices in this arena.

As we speak, sixty percent of the children heading into the batter's box may strike out, partially, because we as parental coaches are more concerned about eating our cultural diet than we are about the impact our dietary choices are having on our home team members. Ethnic food is crippling our future athletes. Ethnic food is guaranteed to reduce our children's earning power, and may cause them to fall into a long term productivity deficit. This fattening food is prematurely killing off the beta cells that produce life sustaining insulin. As parents we can remove it from our homes.

Dianomics plainly lays out the statistics detailing this dire situation. As explained, home centered interventions, and incentives, can win this part of the game for the family. Incentives can unite a family around common goals and redirect our actions and thinking away from our ethnic indulgences. These incentives include intrinsic rewards, like regular praise, and recognition for health behaviors such as avoiding sugared drinks and fattening desserts. These incentives also include extrinsic financial rewards such as weakly allowances tied to an hour of daily physical activity and proper meal choices. This is what home base is all about. It is about winning at our own game.

The family, with the parent as coach, offers the pristine environment for nurturing greater physical activity, while strengthening one another in our healthy eating choices. The parent is able to create and manage incentives that are free from bureaucratic haggling, free from unneeded legislation, and free from excessive outside interference. As parent coaches, we can go to a man-to-man offense, tailor our interventions, create just the right emphasis, and call upon the resources of the team owners. For at-risk children we can walk together with them to school, and walk into the office where kids are weighed. We can get on the scale first. If by some odd chance we end up with feedback that surprises us, by standing on that scale, we can immediately engage the solutions. We can be prepared to hit a home run. We can see our physicians and start on a treatment plan that includes incentives.

Ladies and Gentlemen

The bases are loaded. The time for action is now. It is the bottom of the ninth inning, and the other team is winning. We have two strikes against us, our examples and our lack of incentives. The odds are slim, but we love slim. We will hit a home run, with the bases loaded, and win the game. This is why:

We have in our favor a free form of government, semi-responsive to citizen advocacy. We have a tremendous health safety net. Currently, Medicaid covers one in five of us with the assistance of our supplemental food program. We have the world's most developed health insurance system covering newborns to centenarians (some 70,000!). We have the best trained physicians and health care workers in the world. Our technology is first rate, with more phenomenal health innovations on the near horizon. We research and test to the nth degree. We basically have the whole package – we are missing only one ingredient: incentives.

You may, by now, rightly consider that I have beaten the incentives message to death. Good – because no one else has tried to put the whole package in front of the general public. No author has made the claim that we can stop diabetes and the death of our beta cells by systematically and ubiquitously inserting incentives into our homes, our food purchases, our taxes, our schools, our companies, our insurance benefits, our state insurance, our senior insurance, our physician reimbursement, our hospital reimbursement, and our pharmaceutical industry. The cure for the diabetes epidemic will not be found in the science of medicine. The cure will be found in the science of economics.

Dianomics further claims that diabetes can be stopped without raising taxes (in total), without raising insurance costs, and without charging our seniors more for their health care. *Dianomics: The Economics of Diabetes*, claims that incentives will drive down costs while increasing the quality of health care. It rests on behavioral economic principles, not medical science and more education. The claims of *Dianomics* rest on the simple premise that we are not motivated enough to change our behavior.

The ability does not yet exist for our healthcare institutions and government bodies to readily make these incentives real and powerful. The ability to make these incentives work to our advantage already resides in each of our personal lives and within our families. This takes us back to home base.

Home is the place where the *Dianomics* revolution can begin. Home is where families may begin to implement the principles discussed in *Dianomics* and celebrate a victory over disease as they succeed in the effort. By implementing *Dianomics* we will hit a home run, and win the prize of a healthy, happy and productive life. See you at the ball park.

Brent W. Robinson

Chapter 10
Reference List

Asch, David A. and Volpp, Kevin G. "Redesigning Employee Health Incentives: Lessons from Behavioral Economics." New England Journal of Medicine 365.5 (2011): 388-390.

Dixon, A. (2008). Motivation and Confidence: What Does It Take To Change Behavior. Retrieved, 12-27-2011 from http://www.kingsfund.org.uk/document.rm?id=8273

ABOUT THE AUTHOR

Brent W. Robinson MBA is President of The Diabetes Economist, Inc. He also serves as Vice President, Customer Experience at the Institute for Health and Productivity Management (www.IHPM.org), where he has been instrumental in creating the IHPM WorkPlace™ Center for Employee Health Incentives. He has 30 years of experience educating patients and providers on how to prevent the complications of diabetes.

Brent is the proud eternal companion to Debbie. They are the happy parents of four beautiful children, two joyfully married, and two grandchildren. He can be reached at: bwrtop@gmail.com.

Please see www. Diaecon.com for additional information.

www.ingramcontent.com/pod-product-compliance
Lightning Source LLC
Chambersburg PA
CBHW071321310526
45789CB00015B/74